Fundamental Textbook for Overseas Students of
Huazhong University of Science & Technology

Essential Theory of Health Management

Chief Editor Fang Pengqian

Deputy Editor Zhang Hongxing

Xiang Fei

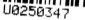

U0250347

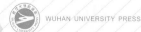
WUHAN UNIVERSITY PRESS

图书在版编目(CIP)数据

健康事业管理概论 = Essential Theory of Health Management/方鹏骞主编.
—武汉:武汉大学出版社,2016.11
ISBN 978-7-307-18719-1

Ⅰ.健… Ⅱ.方… Ⅲ.卫生管理学—医学院校—教材 Ⅳ.R19

中国版本图书馆 CIP 数据核字(2016)第 235264 号

责任编辑:胡 艳 责任校对:汪欣怡 版式设计:韩闻锦

出版发行:**武汉大学出版社** (430072 武昌 珞珈山)
(电子邮件:cbs22@whu.edu.cn 网址:www.wdp.com.cn)
印刷:武汉中科兴业印务有限公司
开本:787×1092 1/16 印张:9.25 字数:216 千字 插页:1
版次:2016 年 11 月第 1 版 2016 年 11 月第 1 次印刷
ISBN 978-7-307-18719-1 定价:28.00 元

Preface

As the deepening of the Reform and Opening-up in China and the improvement of China's international status, the importance of the globalisation of education has reached a new level. *National Medium and Long-term Educational Reform and Development Program* (2010—2020) points out that we must reinforce communication and cooperation with foreign counterparty so as to improve the globalisation process of our education. In order to enhance our nation's international education system, it is critical that we build a foreign students service system which matches our international status and education demand. To achieve this, the Ministry of Education published the *Schedule for Studying in China* and aimed to become the biggest studying destination in Asia.

Huazhong University of Science & Technology is under the direct administration of the Ministry of Education, and is one of the top universities in China. It is imminent for our university to build an education model that cultivates foreign students that reflect our standard of education. To achieve this, we need the curricular system and textbooks that are of international standards. At present, our university has approximately 3600 foreign students who come from more than 130 countries around the world. Most of them attend medical majors and, therefore, the quality of the curricular system, textbooks and reference materials for medical foreign students will largely decide the level of international education of our university. Clinical medicine and public health deal with individual and group health respectively, while health management aims to improve health development for the whole society. This is why, based on teaching experience of many years, Professor Fang Pengqian from Huazhong University of Science & Technology and his team design this textbook specifically for foreign medical students in our university.

Health management focuses on the development of medical and health care industry and has a unique knowledge structure and specific methodologies. This interdisciplinary subject examines the problems in the development of heath care industry from various perspectives and utilises knowledge from Management, Politics, Economics, Sociology and Ethics. Usually, what confuse medical students are not only clinical related problems, but also issues related to medical insurance, health system, hospital management. Therefore, this book is crucial for medical students as it helps them develop problem-solving abilities in this field.

Essential Theory of Health Management is a core course for medical foreign students. On the one hand, it is a crucial textbook for foreign students majored in Clinical Medicine, Preventive Medicine, Nursing Science and so on, while it also is an important reference book for foreign students of other majors. On the other hand, this book is suitable for Chinese students who are interested in interpreting health management problems from an international perspective.

This is the first English textbook on health management that is designed for foreign medical students in our university. This book illustrates both theoretical and practical issues about health management organisations, public health management, community health management, costs of clinical treatments, hospital information system and hospital resource planning, and includes case studies of national and international affairs.

Professor Fang is well-known for his contributions to the health management field and has focused his research on medical and health industry reform, hospital management, global health issues. Meanwhile, Professor Fang is well-respected for his rich teaching experience on the medical and health industry reform in China. Professor Fang always actively seeks feedback from foreign students and pays great attention to their needs and interests. Thus, I firmly believe that this book is a must-have for those who want to learn about health management and will contribute tremendously to our university's education system for foreign medical students.

Contents

Contents

Chapter 1　Introduction

1.1　Summary of Management

1.1.1　Concept of Management

Many experts and scholars made different interpretations of management from different perspectives. Some representative views are as follows:

Frederick Winslow Taylor, the founder of scientific management theory, thought management to know exactly what you want the workers to do, and then make them use the best and the most economical way to complete it. This shows that management a clear goal, is to teach employees the methods of work, in order to achieve the goal in the best way.

Henri Fayol, the founder of the modern management theory, raised one of the first comprehensive statements of a general theory of management. He proposed that there were five primary functions of management and fourteen principles of management.

Harold Koontz, a professor of California University in Los Angeles, said that management is to design and maintain a good environment which makes people in the group to achieve the goal of high efficiency.

Simon Herbert believed that management is decision-making. Although this definition fails to reflect the content of management, it highlights the dominant position of decision-making in management, and emphasizes the decision-making is throughout the process of management, which indicates the inner relationship between the decision and management.

American management scientist Stephen P. Robbins said that management refers to the process of being more effective with others, or through other people's activities.

Some scholars in our country also give some definitions, such as Zhang Shangren said that management is the technology, science and activities which the organization and people control itself to achieve goals.

The so-called management is the process of integrating the resources of the organization effectively through the planning, organizing, leading, controlling and other activities in order to achieve the goal in the specific environment. It contains the following four meanings:

(1) As a purposeful activity of an organization, management must aim at the organization's goal. It is a conscious and purposeful process.

（2）Management should be reflected and completed through the planning, organizing, leading, controlling and other activities, but they are just part of the means or methods to help effectively integrate resources.

（3）The emphasis of management is on the effective integration of organizational resources (including human, finance, material, information, technology, time, reputation, etc.).

（4）Management activities are performed in a certain environment. Environment has created certain conditions and opportunities, but also poses certain constraints and threats. Effective management must take into account the specific conditions from internal and external organization.

1.1.2　Functions of Management

In order to accomplish the management task, the role of the management functions needs to be played. The most commonly cited functions of management are planning, organizing, leading, and controlling, despite the fact that some identify additional functions.

（1）Planning is the function of management that involves setting objectives and determining a course of action for achieving these goals. Planning determines the direction of the whole organization, and is the primary function of management. Management activities in the logical order always start with planning. Organizing, leading and controlling must follow the planning. Therefore, in a broad sense, they belong to the implementation of planning. Generally speaking, the program and the contents of planning mainly include the following three aspects:

① Environmental scanning: Planners must be aware of the critical contingencies that their organization faces, in terms of economic conditions, their competitors and their customers. Planners need to forecast future conditions. These forecasts are the basis for planning.

② Decision making: Based on external environment and internal conditions, according to the opportunities and threats that may be offered in the environmental change, and the resources' advantages and weaknesses of the organization, it must choose the direction, goal and path of future actions. Decision making is especially important in the planning stage, despite the fact that it is throughout the whole process of management. It determines the quality of the plan, and determines the level of the entire management.

③ Developing action plans: Planners must establish objectives, the statements of what needs to be achieved and when. Planners must identify alternative courses of action for achieving objectives. After evaluating the various alternatives, planners must make decisions about the best courses of action for achieving objectives. They must formulate the necessary steps and ensure effective implementation of plans. Finally, planners must constantly evaluate the performance of their plans and take corrective measures when it's necessary.

（2）Organizing is the function of management that involves developing an organizational structure and allocates the human resources to guarantee the accomplishment of objectives. The structure of the organization is the framework within which the effort is coordinated. The structure is usually represented by an organization chart, which provides a graphic representation of the chain of command within an organization. The specific procedures and contents of the organizing include three parts: organizational design, staffing, and organizational change.

① Organization design: According to the plan, it will set up the positions. According to a certain standard, it will combine these positions, and form into different departments. And according to the organizational and environmental characteristics, it will determine the relationship among the different departments.

② Staffing: According to the requirements of each job activity as well as the quality and skill characteristics of organization members, it will select the appropriate placement in the relevant post, make appropriate work that will be borne by the right people.

③ Organizational change: According to the changes in the organization and its environment, the adjustment of the organization and structure is necessary. It can eliminate the aging condition of the organization, overcome organizational inertia, optimize the allocation of resources, and realize the dynamic balance between human and business in the organization. It can also assure the organization's vitality, and to achieve organizational goals effectively.

(3) Leading is the third function of management. Working under this function helps the management control and supervise the staff. It also gives them the opportunity to render assistance to the employees by guiding them to the right direction, to achieve the company's goals and also accomplish their personal or career goals, which can be powered by motivation, communication, department dynamics, and department leadership.

Leading attempts to motivate and lead the employees toward the planned objectives. It aims to delegate tasks to subordinates, the right approach to it can be helpful to increasing the productivity of the entire organization. Leading is an anthropological function of management, and that deals with people on a personal basis. Managers who have the responsibility to lead the staff have to be sensitive to behavior patterns and have the ability to read body language so as to make more informed decisions regarding their workers.

(4) Controlling, the last step of the management functions, which includes the establishing performance standards, which balancing the company's objectives. It also involves evaluation and reporting of actual job performance. When these points are studied by the management, it is necessary in order to compare all these things. This study or comparison leads to further corrective and preventive actions. The controlling function aims to confirm that if the tasks being allotted are performed in time and in accordance with the standards set by the quality department.

Controlling happens after the planning process has been put in place and the tasks assigned. It aims to see if the results are consistent with the objectives set forth in the original plan. Standards must be adjusted according to the available resources and accounting for external factors which may affect performance. The controlling process, in comparison with the other three, is a continuous process. All levels of management take part in this function. Control is also dynamic in nature as the management can anticipate future problems, adopt necessary prophylactic measures, and make policy changes in time.

The management functions of planning, organizing, leading, and controlling are widely regarded as the best means of describing the manager's job as well as the best way to classify accumulated knowledge about the study of management. Despite the fact that there have been tremendous changes in the environment faced by managers and the tools used by managers to perform their roles, managers still perform these essential functions.

1.1.3 Characteristics of Management

Management is a dynamic and creative activity, which can effectively integrate the resources of the organization in order to achieve the goal of the organization. Such activity is different from cultural activity, scientific activity and educational activity.

1.1.3.1 Is Management a Social Phenomenon or Cultural Phenomenon

As long as there is a human society, there is management. As long as it is common for many people (i.e., to a common goal), it is needed in order to achieve the benefits of collaboration by making plans and setting goals and other activities. Therefore, management is a social phenomenon or a cultural phenomenon. Two basic conditions for the existence of management are that there must be two people at least in the collective activity, and there must be a consistent goal.

1.1.3.2 The Carrier of Management Is Organization

Many of the activities of management are carried out in a certain organization. There is no management without an organization. Therefore, the carrier of management is the organization.

1.1.3.3 The Core of Management Is to Deal with All Kinds of Relationships

Management does not constitute an individual activity; it is implemented in a certain organization. Everything in the organization is communicated and handled by the person, so the manager is indeed in charge of the employees. Management activities need to deal with people from the beginning to the end. Therefore, the core of management is tantamount to dealing with all kinds of relationships.

1.1.3.4 Scientificalness and Artistry of Management

Management activities should follow the requirements of the scientific management in the process of objective laws, and embody the art of contingency requirements. This is the scientificalness and artistry of management.

1. Scientificalness of Management

As an active process, there are a series of basic objective laws in management. After numerous failures and successes, people summed up a series of management theories and general methods by collecting, summarizing and detecting the data in the practice, putting forward the hypothesis, verifying hypothesis. People use these theories and methods to guide their management practices, and utilize the results of management activities to measure the management of the theories and methods that used in the process whether it is effective or correct. Management of scientific theories and methods in practice has been verified and enriched. Management is a science, which reflects the management theories and methods of the empirical law, and has a set of scientific methods to analyze and solve problems.

2. Artistry of Management

Management must be built on the environment and change, pay attention to the way, and avoid mechanical management. Management is an art, any manager must put forward the corresponding countermeasures according to current situation. Sometimes the failure happens, mainly because of the regardless of the actual situation and the neglect of the artistry of management.

3. The Relationship Between the Scientificalness and Artistry of Management

The scientificalness and artistry of management are interdependent and complementary to each other. The systematic nature of management reveals the rules of management activities, and reflects the common characteristics of management; the artistry of management is to reveal the special rules of management, and reflect the personality of management. The generic characters exist in the personality, that is, the scientific nature of management is included in different management practices. Each management activity is not only the usual requirements of management, but also their own characteristics.

The scientificalness and artistry of management interact with each other. The former lays the foundation for the latter, which enables the manager to grasp the essence of management, and thus has a steady stream of creativity; the latter is to make the management complete from theory to practice, from abstract to concrete, and be flexible in all kinds of situations.

Understanding management is the unity of science and art, which enables the manager to realize the organic combination of scientific management and the management of art. It is advantageous for the manager to realize the management effectively.

1.2 Health Services

1.2.1 The Conception of Social System and Health System

1.2.1.1 Social System

In the book *General System Theory: Foundations, Development and Applications*, American biologist L.V. Bertalanffy, who is the founder of system theory pointed out that the system is a number of elements in accordance with the specific structure, each links with a specific function of the whole body. The system structure consists of the relationship among the elements, structure determines the system function. According to the hierarchical division, the social system in the world can be divided into different regions and countries, for the nation, it is divided into different industries; for the industry, it is subdivided into different enterprises, units, institutions or families; for the enterprises and units, it is divided into different departments; it is eventually settled into the natural person (the basic elements of social systems). Social systems are generally divided into other subsystems (such as education, health, science, technology, etc.) in the economic, political, cultural, ecological and social systems.

1.2.1.2   Health System

Health system includes the organizations, institutions and resources aimed at developing health activity for the purpose of promoting, recovering and maintaining health. The key words of the definition are "health activity", whether it is private health care or public health service, or the health promotion activity with several departments, as long as the intention is to promote, recover or maintain health, then it can be considered as health activity, which means, the judgment standard of health activity is that whether the original starting point aimed at promoting, recovering or maintaining health. For example, improving the nutritional status of residents, improving the level of population education and so on, these are conducive to the improvement of health, but if the original starting point of the improvement of nutritional status and education level is not from a point of health view, but from the others, it can not be called health activity.

Health system is a complex system, any individuals, groups, organizations and related resources that take promoting, recovering and maintaining of health as the main goal are within the category. Such as preventive health care and medical service providers, funding agencies, producers of medicine, reagents and medical equipments, doctors and nurses, managers and planners of health service, etc.. Thus, health system has the characteristics of multi-participation. All aspects of this system are interrelated and interacted with each other, and they need to work together to achieve the ultimate goal of the system.

From the viewpoint of system theory, first of all, the health system is an organic circle, the function of the health system is greater than the sum function of each subsystem. Secondly, the subsystems of the health system are not isolated. At the same time, the elements and subsystems are interrelated, which constitute the indivisible unity of the health system.

1.2.2   The Function and Influence of Social System on Health System

From the view of the social system, as a subsystem of the social system, the health system can realize the best function of the social system only by the coordinated and balanced development of other subsystems of society. The specific effects and functions of other subsystems on the health system are as follows:

1.2.2.1 Economic System

The level and strategy of national economic development determine the amount of the investment quota and available resources in the process of health development. The higher the cost of investing in health, the more resources to improve the providing of health services .

1.2.2.2 Political System

In a country, the internal political environment and the ruling party's intention, affect the direction and goal of the health development, as well as the height and position of health problems in social development. In the early stages of development, the ruling party is more inclined to "take economic construction as the center", neglect the importance of health in the national economy for a short period. However, in the developed countries, especially the welfare oriented countries, such as the United Kingdom, Sweden, and so on, usually place the health in the important position of social development.

1.2.2.3 Cultural System

Cultural environment is related to the residents' values of health or ethics in a country or region. The effects of cultural environment on the health are mainly shown in the following three aspects: the overall value of the society, the medical personnel's practice concepts, and the health expectations of people. In addition, from the perspective of the demand and supply of economics, the growing demands of health are inexhaustible power to promote the development of health service.

1.2.2.4 Ecosystem

Ecosystem provides material support for the development of health system. Health system is based on the ecological system, the building materials, the raw medicine materials of health organization, and even the air, water resources which medical personnel rely on to survive are provided by ecosystem. In addition, the changes of the ecosystem affect the risk of disease. If the ecosystem is polluted and destroyed, it will lead to disease.

1.2.2.5 Other Subsystems

The other subsystems in the social system mainly affect the structure and quality of the population, the level of science and technology and so on. The population quality and structure determine the characteristics of the disease spectrum, and then affect the development of health.

1.2.3   Functions of Health System

The functional frame of health system includes the following four aspects:

(1) providing health services;

(2) providing medical support, including financing to establish a pool of funds, the allocation of funds for the purchase of services;

(3) raising resources, including human resources, material resources and financial resources;

(4) management, the health system acts as a housekeeper, manage funds, allocate power, and respond to the expectations of people.

Figure 1-1 shows the relations between functions and objectives of health system.

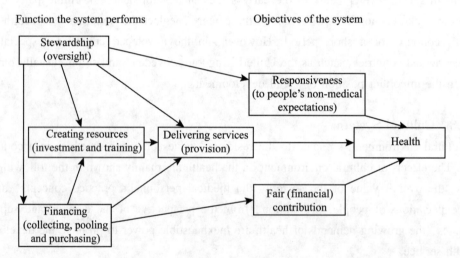

Figure 1-1   Relations between Functions and Objectives of Health System

1.2.3.1   Providing Health Services

Health services include medical services and public health services, mainly cover the medical, prevention, health care, rehabilitation, family planning, infectious diseases prevention and controlling. Providing health services is the core function of the health system, but under different political and economic systems and population conditions, the focus of health services are not the same. The low income and less developed countries focus on the prevention and control of infectious diseases (such as malaria, AIDS, etc.). In the developed countries, the patterns and contents of health services provision have been changed from acute non-communicable diseases to chronic non communicable diseases gradually.

1.2.3.2   Providing Medical Support

Providing health support in health system cover the following three aspects:

(1) Financing: medical insurance funds mainly come from 3 channels (government, society and individual), the individual payment proportion and catastrophic health expenditure incidence are closely linked with the poverty occurred rate due to illness.

(2) Establishing capital pool: coordinate the funds. Improving the overall level is the necessary measures to enhance the ability to adjust the fund, reduce the gap in the structure of funds, and enhance the ability to resist risks.

(3) The provision and purchase of services: the government should take into account, the health care needs of residents, as well as the impacts of different purchase programmes on health outcomes, and consider the cost effectiveness.

1.2.3.3   Raising resources

Total health cost is total health funds available in a country. To determine the total health cost, the national development strategy and the social development goals in a short period of time should be considered comprehensively. Health resources can be raised by the health system, which can be influenced by the health personnel training, health institutions' constructions and medical technology development.

1.2.3.4   Management

Management plays a special role in the functional location of health system, which is not only directly acting on the other 3 functions, but also has direct or indirect effects on all results. Management work includes building the operating rules, the strategic direction of health system, in order to promote the elements of the health system which carry out activities in accordance with the overall objectives.

1.2.4   Characteristics of Health System

1.2.4.1   The General Characteristics

Health system is open and complex. Firstly, the health system and the external political environment, economic environment and natural conditions are inextricably linked. National political system and macroeconomic policy determine the overall direction of the health system, while external human recources, material resources and other resources affect the resource structure and configuration of the health system. The epidemic and outbreak of disease also determine the key and emergency mode of health system. Secondly, the health system is not a single simplified system, its internal system interacts with each other. Drug supply system, medical security system, health service supply system build association through the formation of materials and informations.

1.2.4.2   The Special Characteristics

The basic goal of the health system is to promote the health of people. Health right is a basic right that people should enjoy, to promote the health of people is the core objective and the fundamental purpose of the health system. Raising the health level of people is not only meaning that residents can obtain medical service in time, but also embodied in the whole process from birth to death, from the cradle to the grave.

The products and services provided by the health system are professional. Human body is a sophisticated and complex system, the prevention of disease, diagnosis, treatment and rehabilitation needs professional technical support. Medical personnel must undergo systematic training and obtain a certain qualification before providing patients with high quality health services. Practice (assistant) physicians, practice (assistant) nurses must pass the national examination, and practice after registration. The products and services provided by the health system have the characteristics of public goods and quasi public goods, which have significant economic benefits and social benefits. Take TB prevention and controlling as an example, the possibility of residents become the source of infection of BCG vaccination has been greatly decreased, reduce the probability of the surrounding residents infected with TB at the same time. In the course of the planned immunization, both the vaccinated and non-vaccinated persons are benefited. From the economic theory, public products are non-competitive and non-exclusive, it is difficult to rely on market mechanism to ensure supply. The external benefit of the quasi public goods also determines the deficiency of supply and demand of the public goods.

Health level has a direct impact on the national economy. The outbreak of the disease is not measurable, the disease risk and the economic burden of the disease are easy to bring about negative influence to the individual, family and society. Human resource is the core of social development, if the quality of human resource is declining, that will affects the economic development. The disease risk possibility would lead to poor families due to illness.

1.3   Health Management

1.3.1   The Concept of Health Management

Health management is all the management affairs the state and society take to prevent and cure diseases, maintain and promote the health of the population. Health management can be divided into macro management, medium management and micro management. Among them, macro management takes the development direction and strategy of the national health service as the main object, and the medium management is the management of the health system and the region.Micro management is the management of the internal operation of medical and health institutions.The health management, which is discussed in this book, is mainly focused on the management of the medium level(see Figure 1-2).

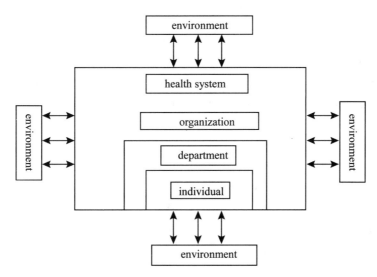

Figure 1-2   The Field of Health Management

1.3.2   The Subject and Object of Health Management

1.3.2.1   The Subject of Health Management

The health management discussed in this book focus on the medium level management, the main body of it includes the following two categories: firstly, government departments and other relevant government departments (such as the development and reform departments, human resources and social security departments, food and drug supervision and management departments, health supervision departments, etc.). Secondly, other social organizations, such as industry associations, societies, etc.

1.3.2.2   The Object of Health Management

The object of health management is that main body's management behavior to achieve management. The object of the health service management includes health organization and its constituent elements and function activities.

(1) Health organization and its constituent elements mainly include: medical service providers, such as hospitals, community health service institutions, village health rooms, private clinics and others; public health service institutions, such as the centers for disease

control and prevention (CDC), blood, tuberculosis prevention, and control institute, organizations of the drug production, circulation and supplement. Constituent elements of the organization mainly include human resources, capital, material equipments, time and information.

(2) Activities carried out by organizations to achieve their functions are the general object of health management. Organizations of management play the function through planning, organizing, leading, controlling. The functional activities of health management include: compiling and carrying out the health plan, health resource allocation, making clear the contents and methods of health services, supervising the health organization and organization behavior, evaluating the performance and optimizing the health policy.

Chapter 2   The Basic Connotation
of Health Management

2.1   Health Development Strategy

2.1.1   The Concept of Health Development Strategy

Health development strategy is based on the needs of health service development and people's health improvement, and it develops global, regular, hierarchical and determined plans for global, long-term, major health problem. Health development strategy is an important area of national economic and social development strategies, and it keeps coordinated with the national economic and social development strategy. Developing health development strategy in line with national conditions is an important part of improving people's health, promoting economic and social development, keeping society harmonious and stable.

2.1.2   Characteristics of Health Development Strategy

2.1.2.1   Global

Global can be called overall. Health development strategy takes the law of overall development of health service as the research object. It directs overall activities of health service, and pursuits the development of health service as a whole. Health development strategy can also include the local activities of health service, but these activities are as integral parts of the overall activities in health development strategy.

2.1.2.2   Long-term

Health development strategy is a long-term planning of health development, related to overall survival and development of health problems. It is focused on the future, based on scientific prediction to seek long-term development of health service, and mainly concerned with long-term benefits of health service.

2.1.2.3   Leading

Health development strategy involves all aspects of health development. It requires the participation and support of the upper and lower managers and all the staff of health-related organizations. The most senior executives involved in the strategic management of the organization are very important, because they are able to take on the overall organizations and fully understand the situation of the organizations.

2.1.2.4 Programmatic

Health development strategy and the determined strategic targets, strategic priorities and strategic countermeasures are directional and principled. Health development strategy is the program of health service development and authoritative guidance for all activities of health service activities. It must be decomposed and implemented, and then translate into concrete action plans.

2.1.2.5 Suitability

Health development strategy should conform to the external environment and internal conditions. In the process of implementation of the strategy, we should adjust it duly to adapt to the changes of the environment and conditions. At the same time, with the possibility of changes and new development opportunities, we should improve the strategy and set new strategy, so as to achieve the development of health goals.

2.1.2.6 Perspective

Health development strategy is geared to the future. The fundamental purpose is to seek long-term survival and development through the management of the uncertainty of health service development. Health service should not only identify the realities of where they are located correctly, but also predict the development trend of the environment effectively. Moreover, the health service should also plan carefully, mobilize all the resources that can be mobilized to influence the direction and pace of environmental change.

2.2   Health Management System

Health management system refers to a country or region at all levels of government and related health organization architecture, institutional settings, affiliation, responsibilities division, etc. It is the subject of the national management of health affairs. The ordered conduction and management efficiency of health management activities will be directly related to the public health insurance and the sustainable development of national economy and society. Health management system is an open system, and its surrounding environment is affected by factors such as the political system, economic system, financial system, the price system, personnel management system.Internal environment also relates to the coordination and division of labor with other related organizations, as well as the transmission of information within the system organization, business regulation, execution of laws and regulations, etc. But its function will only be reflected in continuous operation, and continue to seek a balance and adaptation environment, and provide better health services for the society. For example, China's current health management system is combination of central and regional system while giving priority to the regional system. Strip refers to industry management system from top to bottom. Block means the provinces (autonomous regions and municipalities), cities (prefecture) and counties, township and other local administrative management.

2.3 Overview of Health Resources Planning

2.3.1 Concept of Health Resources

"Health resources" refers to the social investment of human, financial and material resources in the field of health services, including health human, costs, facilities, equipments, drugs, knowledge and technology, etc. It refers to the certain social economy condition of the state, the collective and individual for comprehensive investment objective reflection of the health care, including the number of health institutions, the number of beds, the number of health personnel, health funds and health funding as a percentage of GDP of a country or region, which are important indicator of health status of a country or a region

Scarcity is a basic characteristic of health resources, there is always a big gap between the actual requirements of the crowd and the health resources provided by the society. The rational allocation of health resources is the basis and prerequisite to provide good health services. Studing the rational allocation of health resources, and improving the allocation of health resources as much as the possibility of fairness and efficiency are the basic tasks of health services research.

There are three kinds of the methods of allocation of health resources: planning configuration method, market allocation method, planning and market regulation combined method.

2.3.2 Planning Configuration Method

Planning configuration method means that the government's mandatory plans and administrative measures as the main way of the allocation of health resources. It reflects the integrity and fairness of health services and avoids the imbalance of resources allocation because of the differences in geography and economic. It is an important means of health resources allocation, also known as macro-configuration.

2.3.3 Market Allocation Method

Market allocation method is to achieve the allocation of health resources in different areas and levels through competition, prices, supply and demand, and other market mechanisms. Market allocation method can reflect efficiency principle, and make the limited health resources allocate to the fields of high efficiency. However, the nature and characteristics of health service decide that the market mechanism will not have a basic configuration effect on health resources, which is reflected that the market mechanism can't solve the problem of the fairness of allocation of health resources.

2.3.4   Planning and Market Regulation Combined Method

Planning and market regulation combined method refers to the way in which the government macroeconomic regulation and control play the guiding role of the planning and adjustment, and supplemented by health resource allocation of market regulation. Planning configuration and market allocation have their advantages and disadvantages. The practice of health service development and health resources allocation domestic and international shows that a single planned regulation or market regulation is not conducive to the effective allocation of health resources. Both of them must be took together and play their strengths, in order to achieve the optimal allocation of resources and promote the health development of health services.

The United Kingdom implements National Health Service(NHS) system. Health funds are mainly mobilized by the government through taxation. The government conducts overall plans of health resources allocation, and directly holds public health institutions, and offers a free or nearly free health care services. There is also a part of the health services by signing a contract, and government purchase the health services from the privates. The basic features are: medical and health care funds raised through taxes, raise funds and main service provider by the government, the funds that government invests are used to reflect the benefits of the social service sector, universal coverage and fairness for access to health care services.

In the management system, the United Kingdom implements centralized and unified management, hospital nationalization, employing the civil servants, general doctors and contract doctors are the basic backbone. Service system is made up of three parts: the primary service, community service and specialized service. Among them, the primary service and community service shall be the responsibility of the general doctors and nurses, and the specialized service is provided by public hospitals. Patients who get to the hospital must be transferred by general practitioners. The most important part of the NHS system is the public hospitals. Public hospitals belong to the government agency or subsidiary, and the staff belong to the state civil servants or government employees.

In the United Kingdom, public hospitals account for about 95% of the total national hospitals. In the 1990s, the Conservative government had tried to introduce the competitive mechanism characterized " internal market" reform to improve efficiency of national health system problems. But then the problems appeared, such as medical service unfairness and the high cost of management, which are criticized by people. After the Labour government came to power in 1997, they canceled the "internal market" reform to emphasize the basic principles of government responsibility, public-private cooperation and social solidarity. In 2003, the health costs of the United Kingdom accounted for 8% of total GDP, the total health expenses per capita was $2428, and was relatively low in developed countries.

2.4 Summary of Health Human Resource Management

2.4.1 The Concept of Health Human Resources and Health Human Resource Management

2.4.1.1 Health Human Resources

Health human resources refer to the workers receiving health education and vocational training, working in the health system, solving the problem of health, providing health services, protecting the public physical and mental health. According to the differences between the service areas, the nature of works and jobs, health human resources can generally be divided into four categories:

(1) Health care professional and technical personnel, including doctors, nurses, pharmacists and imaging personnel, etc.

(2) Health managers, that can be divided into health service managers and health administrators. The former is mainly engaged in health care, disease control, health surveillance, food inspection, medical education and scientific research, etc. The latter is mainly engaged in the personnel, finance, information work, etc.

(3) Skill workers and service personnel, that mainly include auxiliary health work tasks of logistics personnel.

(4) Other health workers, such as community health workers.

2.4.1.2 Health Human Resource Management

Health human resource management is giving full play to people's initiative and creativity, to serve the public health development and achieve health system goals, using modern scientific system, laws, methods and procedures, respecting a reasonable human resource for health planning, training, organization, coordination, control and incentives, and performance evaluation of continuous dynamic management process. Health system is a knowledge and technology intensive industry. It is also a labor-intensive industry. It is a complex network system of division of labor cooperation. Thus the knowledge, skills and attitudes of health service staff to improve the quality and level of health care play a decisive role, health human resource configuration optimization is essential for the overall health system performance and output.

2.4.2   The Basic Content of Health Human Resource Management

Health human resource management is throughout the entire health human resources for movement. It includes quantity, quality, structure, hierarchy, distribution and flow management of health human resource, and also includes health human resource for health planning, access, authentication, use and performance evaluation management.

A certain quantity and quality of health human resource is the foundation of the health system operation. The structure, geographical distribution and hierarchical relationship of the health human resource are related to the key to the scientific and reasonable configuration of health human resource in the health system. Meanwhile, the health care system itself is a dynamic system that requires constant adjustments. The flow of health human resource is an important means to adjust the structure of health human resource and scientific, reasonable and rational distribution.

However, in order to achieve a reasonable number, size, structure and balanced configuration of health system, we need to implement the health human resource planning management, the access and authentication management health human resource, health human resource allocation management, health human resource development management, the flow of health human resource management, health human resource for compensation system design and performance evaluation management. As a result, quantity, quality, scale, structure and distribution of management and health human resource planning, access, development, compensation, performance evaluation are content of health human resource management system. It reflects the unified of content and process of health human resource management and it also highlights the rich connotation of health human resource management and scientific process of continuous operation, as shown in Figure 2-1.

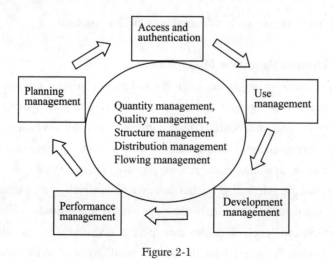

Figure 2-1

2.5 Medical Services Management Overview

2.5.1 Medical Services

2.5.1.1 Concept of Medical Services

Medical services are collectively general term of diagnosis, treatment, rehabilitation and other services. They are provided by various medical institutions at all levels of their medical staff through using a variety of health resources. The body of medical services are various medical institutions at all levels and its medical staff; the object of medical services is the majority of the public, mainly the people who are suffering from various diseases and in a state of subhealthy; the contents of medical services include diagnosis, treatments and rehabilitation services; the purpose of medical services is to protect public health, improve worker productivity and promote the development of social production through providing security, effective and convenient medical services for the public.

With the evolution of the medical model, modern medical services have been expanded from the inside hospital to the outside hospital, which is forming a concept of integrated care. As a service product, medical services at least consist of three levels:

(1) core services, also known as the main services or essential services, are the reason why service products exist, and also the distinction between medical institutions and other institutions.

(2) Form services, namely the form of medical care. That is the quality of care entity.

(3) Ancillary services, increasing the value of the services or distinguishing the services provided by one organization from other competitors.

2.5.1.2 Characteristics of Medical Services

Medical service is a special class of service which is provided to protect the life and health of the public. Medical services not only have the common character of service industry, but also have the particularity of the medical industry. The following aspects are the main features of medical services:

(1) Intangibility. Intangible nature of medical services is the most significant feature. Medical services in essence are an act, process and performance, which is different from tangible products provided by production enterprises. With respect to tangible products, medical services are invisible and intangible. Consumers purchase intangible services, instead of getting a tangible product.

(2) Inseparability. It means that the production and consumption process of medical services occur at the same time. Medical service is a one to one service. The production and

consumption process are consistent in the time and place.

(3) Not to be stored. The feature of medical services is the inevitable extension of inseparability. Medical services are not the tangible products, which can not be stored, repaired or reworked. This feature requires that the service capacity of medical institutions should be applied to the timely treatment services. If not, there is no value, it means the loss and waste of resources.

(4) Public welfare and ethic. Health is a fundamental human right. Chinese health service is a social welfare with a certain welfare nature, which determines the welfare of medical services. Ethics of medical services on the one hand reflects the fact that it is difficult for patients to make scientific judgments about their medical needs and services, so that they have to rely on medical professionals. On the other hand, the patient's privacy, secret parts of the body are exposed to the medical staff. So it is necessary that medical personnel should have noble technical level and lofty professional ethics.

(5) Difference. Difference means that the constituent and quality levels of medical services change frequently, which can not be standardized as tangible things. The utility of every medical services to consumers and consumers' perception of service quality are likely to differ. The medical services provided by the different medical staff of the same medical institution also differ. The require of different patients' who are suffering from the same disease will be different.

(6) High risk. There is a wide range of diseases and patients' condition varies frequently. Any medical behavior is closely related to human life and health. So the medical service industry is a high risk industry. Medical activities must be strictly regulated and the corresponding technical rule should be seriously implemented.

(7) Randomness and continuity. It is difficult to predict when people get sick, what diseases people get, when epidemic happens, and how large epidemic is. So the demand and supply of medical services are not like ordinary daily consumer goods which can be consumed in a plan. It also cannot be mass production according to standard procedures. Medical institutions stress that time is life. They must be available 24 hours a day.

(8) Difficult to monitor and evaluate. Outputs of medical institutions which include social benefits can not be evaluated by a single indicator (such as profit maximization). It is very difficult for both consumers and administration of medical institutions to supervise medical services. The ideal output index of the medical institution is making the people's health level have great improvement with less investment.

(9) Professional. Medical service is highly professional. Medical and health technical personnel should not only obtain the corresponding qualification, but also explain highly professional knowledge to the patient and gain their cooperation and support. The damage to the health of people which is brought by low quality or inappropriate medical services is irreversible and even permanent.

（10）The special nature of the doctor-patient relationship. Doctor-patient relationship is different from the general relationships. In the medical services, because of injury or disease, patients always are in a particular state. And medical institutions gain the initiative in health care, which makes that doctor-patient relationship has become more subtle.

2.5.2 Medical Services Management

2.5.2.1 The Concept of Medical Services Management

Medical services management refers to the progress that government, the laws and regulations related to social health care implement management and supervision to various medical institutions at all levels, health professional and technical personnel, provision of medical services to ensure the quality of medical services and health safety. Medical services management mainly reflects in four aspects:

（1）The management of medical institutions at all levels;

（2）The management of various medical health professional and technical personnel;

（3）The management of the medical services;

（4）The management of various health organizations and their activities.

2.5.2.2 Principles of Medical Services Management

The basic principles of medical services management show as the following:

（1）Correctly handle the relationship between social benefits and economic benefits. Medical service management should insist on the tenet of service for people, give priority to social benefits and prevent one-sided pursuit of economic benefits and ignorance of social benefits. And the management stresses the improvement of the health of residents , gives priority to the development of basic health services and gradually meets the diverse health needs of residents.

（2）Fairness principles. We should make full use of existing medical resources for all people according to the local medical supply and demand. The size of city medical institutions should be properly controlled to ensure that the entire population, especially our rural residents have access to basic medical services.

（3）Accessibility principles. The service radius of medical institutions is appropriate, the transportation is convenient, the layout of medical institutions is rational, which is convenient for the mass to make use of medical services.

（4）The principle of classification. According to the function, task, scale of medical institutions, they can be divided into different levels. It is very important to establish and perfect the medical service of grading medical, two-way referral system. The diagnosis of common diseases, frequently-occurring diseases should be in the medical institutions at grassroots level, while the diagnosis and treatment of emergency and severe cases should be in the urban hospitals.

（5）Public ownership dominant principles. We should adhere to the principle of non-profit medical institutions as the mainstay and profit medical institutions as the supplement. Social capital should be encouraged and guided to promote the development of medical services in order to form the medical system of investment diversification.

（6）The principle of equal emphasis on Chinese and Western medicine. In accordance with the health care policy, Chinese and Western medicine should be paid equal attention. And the development of traditional Chinese medicine should be ensured. There should be a reasonable layout of national medical establishment and the allocation of resources.

（7）The overall benefit principle. Establishment of medical institutions should be in accordance with the requirements of the overall and regional health care planning. We should build a health care system that medical institutions at all levels can coordinate and orderly compete. The local should obey the global. We should make scientific and rational allocation of medical resources to give full play to the overall functionality and efficiency of the health care system.

2.6   Public Health Service Management Overview

2.6.1   Concept of Public Health

The definition of public health varies with different agencies, experts and scholars. There are some more representative definition which are as the following:

Winslow, 1920, one of the leaders of public health in United States, also a professor of Yale University, has given the classic definition that: "Public health is the science and practice to prevent disease, prolong life and improve health. Public health improve environmental health conditions, control epidemic diseases, educate everyone to develop good health habits through organized community action. Health care power can be organized by public health for early diagnosis of the disease and preventive treatment, which can entitle each community member to have healthy bodies to maintain living standards. "Protection of public health is the mission of public health, whose goal is to create a healthy community environment and make people live healthy. The definition of Winslow is summarized as follows: Public health is the science and technology to prevent disease, prolong life, promote health and improve the effectiveness through organized community efforts. As a public health leader in the US, the definition of Winslow is the most influential one in academic area, which is a summary and conclusion of the US public health practice at that time. It also defines the nature, scope and purpose of public health. This definition was adopted by WHO.

In November 1986, WHO convened the first conference on Health Promotion in Ottawa,

Canada and published the famous *Ottawa Charter for Health Promotion*. The meeting proposed the new definition of public health: all activities which are aiming at protecting the population from disease and promoting public health under the leadership of the government and at the level of community. The basic condition of health is peace, shelter, education, food, income, stable environment, sustainable resources, social justice and equality. The core content of public health stresses the core status of the government in public health and puts greater emphasis on the role of social science to promote health.

In 2009, the Chinese medical association held the first national conference on public health in Beijing. The conference puts forward the "Chinese version" definition of public health: public health is the public sector which is for the purpose of guarantee and promotion of public health. Public health aims at controlling diseases and disability, improving the health related to natural and social environment, providing basic medical and health services, cultivating public health literacy, realizing the health promotion of the whole society, creating a society that everyone enjoys a healthy condition through joint efforts of the state and society.

2.6.2 Public Health Service

2.6.2.1 Concept of Public Health Service

Public health service is the product or service provided by the public health department or other organization aiming at protecting the public health and meeting public health needs.

Public service is the core concept of public administration and government reform, including strengthening urban and rural public facilities, the development of science and technology, education, culture, sports, health and other public utilities, providing protection for the public to participate in social, political, economic and cultural activities. Public service emphasizes cooperation, government services and the rights of citizens.

Basic public services are built on the basis of a certain social consensus and development stage and the overall level of social economic. Basic public services aim at maintaining social economic stability and basic social justice and cohesion, protecting the basic right to life and development, achieving the required basic social conditions for the comprehensive development of people. Basic public services are including three basic points: (1) protecting the basic human right to life (or basic survival needs). It requires the government and society provide everyone with basic employment security, basic endowment insurance, basic life guarantee, etc.; (2) meeting the basic dignity (or decent). It requires the government and community provide everyone with basic education and cultural services; (3) meeting the basic health needs. It requires the government and community provide everyone with basic health care for everyone.

2.6.2.2 Characteristics of Public Health Service

Public health service not only has the characteristics of public service, but also has the characteristic of health service. The essential characteristic of public health service is publicity. Publicity is embodied in the following respects:

(1) Public. The beneficiaries of the public health service are the all public.

(2) The commonality. The content of public health service involves the common needs of all the community members.

(3) The public welfare. The goal of public health service is to achieve the common interests of the public and to influence members of community in public life.

(4) Fairness. Public health involves the basic rights of citizens, rather than a mere commodity.

2.6.3   Public Health Management

2.6.3.1   Concept of Public Health Management

Public health management is government-led public health service providers deliver public health services to the community timely and effectively in order to achieve the public interest, and optimize the allocation of public health resources. Public health management also manages the public health system, systematic activities and social measures. Public health management aims at improving natural environment, social environment and promoting human health. It is established as a set of social institutions for the purpose of disease prevention, pain control and improvement of people's health. Public health management includes management of disease control and health supervision. Public health management aims at emphasizing the management responsibility of health administrative organization from the government level. It implements its abilities through all levels of disease prevention institutions and health supervision agencies. The research object of public health management focuses on public health policy, public health organizations, evaluation of public health, public health resources and public health service system.

2.6.3.2   Public Health Service Management

Public health service management is based on the functions and features of public health management, the government implements management of the public health organizational system, system activities and social measures in order to safeguard public health. Public health service management focuses on the rational allocation of public health services resources and the improvement of healthy level of residents and their life quality. While, public health management focuses on public health policy, public health organizations, the planning and evaluation of public health.

2.6.4   The Providers of Public Health Service

The providers of public health service mainly refer to the public, private and voluntary organizations, which can provide the essential public health services within certain scope of competence. The organizations include all levels of government departments, the public health administrations, providers of public health service and health care service, public health academic institutions, communities, enterprises, employers and the media. Public health administrative departments include the departments for disease control and prevention, health supervision, public health emergency and so on, which belong to the national health and family planning commission. And the local health administration such as province, city and county (district) set up the corresponding organs at all levels. The providers of public health services include disease prevention and control, and health monitoring bodies which are established from the national to the local; and various public health research institutes, include public health education and research institutions, the Chinese preventive medical association which are affiliated with all levels of education and health administrative departments and the corresponding association at provincial and municipal levels.

2.6.5 The Management of the Process that Public Health Services Are Provided

The public health services of providing stands for the process that we provide high quality of public health services to all the residents and do our best to safeguard and promote residents' health according to national laws, regulations and policies, using the theory and methods of management science, according to the national economic and social development, the need of disease control, the residents' demand for public health services. The management of the process that public health services are provided mainly includes the management of disease prevention and control, management of health supervision, the management of emergency public health event and health management, etc. In our country, the management is implemented by disease control institutions, health supervision institutions, urban and rural grassroots health service agencies.

2.7 Community Health Service Management

Community health service management is the dynamic creative activities which the plan, organize, lead, control and coordinate the development, distribution and utilization of community health resources, manage scientifically the process of community health service, to achieve the fixed goal and responsibility of community health service. The purpose of community health service management is to solve the main community health problems, meet the basic health services demand of community residents, improve the health level of community residents.

Community health service management is the management process which is based on the community health service. The process of community health service is the service process for the health management of community residents. The basic contents of community health service are basic medical care and public health. The basic characteristics are as follows: primary health care, health centered service, personalized care, integrated care, continuous services, coordinating services, accessibility services, home-based services, community-based services, the working manner of precaution and teamwork. Community health service management is a scientific management process with centring on the basic contents of community health service, and following the basic characteristics of community health service.

2.8　The Theory of Health Systems Performance Assessment

2.8.1　Basic Concepts

The essence of health systems performance is the realization degree of system objectives. Now the definition of health systems performance has not only been confined to the realization degree of goals, but the maintaining level of three goals under the existing resources. In other words, health systems performance is the realization degree of health system goals under the given health resources. That is to say, health systems performance is the realization degree of three total goals that a country's health system has the responsibility to bear under the given health resources.

2.8.2　The Framework of Health Systems Performance Assessment

The purpose of health systems performance assessment is to enhance the ability of decision makers by providing relevant policies and reliable information about the development of health systems; to improve the ability of the public by providing the information of improved health. In most countries, the policy makers and the public are extremely concerned about the domestic and foreign health systems performance: Will our country's health system be able to run well? Why some countries' health systems performance is good, while others not? Why their health system sperformance also have bigger differences even in states with similar health resources? In order to effectively solve these problems and challenges, countries around the world and international organizations are actively exploring.

2.8.2.1　The Framework of International Health Systems Performance Assessment

The WHO is straight committed to develop the systematic method which can be compared between vertical and horizontal to monitor health performance from country to country. In 2000, the WHO decided to put *Health Systems : Improving Performance* as the theme of world health report 2000, also as one of the four strategic direction, so as to attract the attention of the members, and put improving performance as the core task of national health reform.

According to the world health report 2000, the framework of health systems performance assessment, includes these basic processes that forming the object of performance assessment, choosing measure and method according to the object, analyzing the factors that affect performance and putting forward suggestions for performance improvement, such as shown in Figure 2-2.

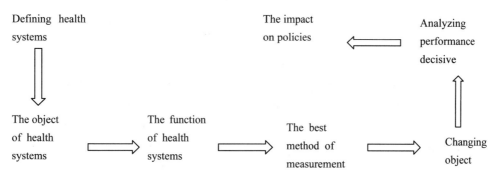

Figure 2-2　The Framework of Health Systems Performance Assessment

Concretely speaking, the health systems performance assessment should include a series of activities:

(1) Measure health systems' contribution to the social expectation object;

(2) Measure health systems and health resources to achieve these goals;

(3) Estimate the efficiency of using these resources to achieve the overall goal;

(4) Assess health systems function, and observe the object and ways of efficiency;

(5) Formulate, carry out policies which can improve the performance and monitor its implementation effect.

According to the goals of the health system, there are five indexes to measure the health system from WHO: the overall level of health; the distribution of health in the population; the overall level of responsiveness; the distribution of responsiveness; and the distribution of financial contribution. When the five indicators are combined by certain proportion, we can conclude a national health system performance. To assess overall population health and thus to judge how well the objective of good health is being achieved, WHO has chosen to use disability-adjusted life expectancy (DALE), which has the advantage of being directly comparable to life expectancy estimated from mortality alone and is readily compared across populations.DALE is estimated from three kinds of information: the fraction of the population surviving to each age group, calculated from birth and death rates; the prevalence of each type of disability at each age group; and the weight assigned to each type of disability, which may or may not vary with age.Survival at each age group is adjusted downward by the sum of all the disability effects, each of which is the product of a weight and the complement of a prevalence (the share of the population not suffering that disability). These adjusted survival shares are then divided by the initial population, before any mortality occurred, to give the average number of equivalent healthy life years that a newborn member of the population could expect to live.

Organisation for economic cooperation and development (OECD) , by reviewing the performance framework and some of the performance indicators adopted recently by WHO , put forward a conceptual framework , including three goals : health improvement , responsiveness to the expectations of consumers and fairness in financial contribution. In addition , there are two types of components for assessment of goal achievement : average level and distribution which are applied to the first two goals (health improvement and responsiveness). Therefore , the framework consists by the measurement indicators from four parts : health promotion and results , responsiveness , equity , and efficiency. This evaluation system was used to evaluate respectively health system performance in Canada , the Netherlands , Sweden , the United Kingdom and the United States. In addition , the World Bank establish the process index system of health systems performance assessment respectively from five key aspects , including financing , payment , organization , regulation and behavior ; and determined the index system of the results of performance assessment index from health conditiion , the financial risk protection and satisfaction.

2.8.2.2   The Framework of Health Systems Performance Assessment of Some Representative Countries

1. The United Kingdom

The United Kingdom established the framework of performance assessment of national health service system in national performance framework. Conceptually , the design of the framework is based on the balanced scorecard. The whole indicators system should have a balance to organizational performance , reflect the main aspects which include the results and the users' view , and should include four aspects : service consumers , internal management , continuous improvement and financial views.

In order to complete the goal , in 1997 , the United Kingdom mainly focused on the following areas : health improvement , equity and accessibility , the effective providing of rational health services. efficiency , patient/caregivers experience , the NHS health outcomes by adopting the new method , through the framework of performance evaluation. In terms of credibility of national health service system , the performance framework mainly includes four aspects : the clinical effectiveness and results , efficiency , the patient/caregivers experience and ability. Under the framework , a series of indicators has be staged that locating widely , such as mental health , cancer treatment , waiting record , the accessibility of family doctors , health , staffing , etc. , and more detailed indicators are staged every year , which is used to assess the performance of the national health service system. The establishment of the framework of performance assessment of national health service is based on the basic health care and communities , these indicators are constant development and improvement as the latest data collection.

2. Australia

Australia gradually established and developed a set of relatively perfect performance framework of health system since the 1990s for guaranteeing the fairness, efficiency and effectiveness of the health system, and clarifying the responsibilities of system in all aspects, which is used for monitoring, evaluating and managing the health system performance. Australia's performance framework of health system reflects and emphasizes the performance of the entire health system, covers the four aspects that are the most important in the medical and health field: population health project, basic health care, medical treatment and the continuity of care services.

Conceptually, the framework based on the model of health determinants, is including three levels: health condition and results, the determinants of health, and health systems performance. There are internal relations between them, for instance, health is affected by the health determinants and health system performance. These three levels are involved fairness problem. It includes four latitudes: health, body function, life expectancy and deaths. The main factors that affect health are mainly to evaluate the factors that affect individual and population health. It includes five dimensions: environment, social economic factors, community, health behavior and other factors related to individual. The framework of health service system performance is to monitor how the health system improves people's health level by improving the quality of medical and health services. The framework consists nine aspects: effectiveness, suitability, efficiency, reactivity, accessibility, safety, consistency, ability and sustainability.

3. Canada

Canadian health service system is a huge, complex system which is mainly on the basis of the public funds system. Under the federal programs, it covers the costs of all hospitals and doctors medical services, including the provinces and autonomous regions. Health systems performance is a part of the Canadian health information indicator framework. The design of the framework mainly answers two questions: The first is the health condition of the Canadian; the second is how the Canada's health service system run. The framework information mainly includes four aspects: health condition, the non-medical determinants of health, health systems performance, the type of community and health system. The latter two test all aspects of the health systems performance by measuring the health services of regional residents. In the framework, the health systems performance includes: acceptability, accessibility, suitability, ability, sustainability, effectiveness, efficiency and security. At present, these areas are indicators except acceptability, ability and sustainability. In health service of community and other types, the indicators are divided into the following categories: community, health systems, and resource. In operational aspects, the framework was promoted through the Canadian institutes of health information network by tracking the health determinants and regional, provincial, national health service.

4. America

American health service system is a distributed system. At the national level, the United States have many developing performance frameworks of health system, including the improvement framework of the national health system which has been put forward, the model of residents' health promotion, the report of national health service quality, the consumer evaluation of health planning study and the data report of health service provider which widely used, non-state performance report. Other documents of performance evaluation include the American management care and the report of the group of quality improvement which is to come by the service centre of (poor residents medical treatment insurance).

The medical research council of America put forward the framework of improving system performance, including six areas: safety, efficacy, patient-centered, sustainability, efficiency and fairness. In 2000, the American government put forward *healthy people in the United States in 2020*, which was based on health determinants and residents health model, and summarized the 28 key areas, put forward 467 goals. In 2003, the report of national health quality put forward the concept of the measurement framework of health system performance, which mainly engaged in two aspects: health service quality, and the demand of medical service of consumers. Health service quality includes: security, effectiveness, patient-centered, sustainability; Consumer health requirements include: to keep healthy, improving, illness or disability, waiting for death. The framework suggested combining the two parts to develop relations in the middle.

Chapter 3　Organization and Management of Primary Health Care

3.1　The Concept of Primary Health Care

3.1.1　Short Definition of Primary Health Care

A cross-disciplinary understanding of Primary Health Care (PHC) acknowledges the role of health care providers from diverse disciplines, within a philosophy and framework of PHC that is guided by the principles of access, equity, essentiality, appropriate technology, multisectoral collaboration, community participation and empowerment.[①] APHC philosophy recognizes that health and health services occur within particular physical environments and their historical, socio-political, economic, and cultural contexts that shape the social determinants of health for individuals, families, groups, communities, regions, or countries.

3.1.2　Conceptual Definition of Primary Health Care

3.1.2.1　Primary Health Care

PHC is a conceptual model which refers to both processes and beliefs about the ways in which health care is structured. PHC encompasses primary care, disease prevention, health promotion, population health, and community development within a holistic framework, with the aim of providing essential community-focused health care.[②] The foundations of PHC are access, equity, essentiality, appropriate technology, multisectoral collaboration, and community participation and empowerment.

3.1.2.2　Primary Care

Primary care is a constituent of PHC: "While primary care is distinct from primary health care, the provision of essential primary care is an integral component of an inclusive primary

---

　　① Unicef, World Health Organization. Primary Health Care: A Joint Report, 1978.

　　② Shoultz J, Hatcher P A. Looking beyond Primary Care to Primary Health Care: An Approach to Community-based Action. Nursing Outlook, 1997, 45(1):23-26.

health care strategy."① The Institute of Medicine describes PHC as: "… the provision of integrated, accessible health care services by clinicians who are accountable for addressing a large majority of personal health care needs, developing a sustained partnership with patients, and practicing in the context of family and community. This definition builds on earlier definitions by the IOM(international organization for migration) and others. It also recognizes the greater complexity of health care delivery in an era of rapid and profound changes—marked by the development of increasingly integrated health care systems—and the greater interdependence of health care professionals in the provision of health services."② The 1978 WHO statement on PHC supports a vision of essential and accessible primary care that meets the personal health needs of individuals and families, as an integral strategy within a comprehensive framework of PHC.

Despite plenty of documents oriented toward defining primary care conclude that "it is in a state of evolution". New definitions of primary care draw upon interdisciplinary perspectives, but there appears to be some consensus that primary care is the first level of contact of individuals and families with the national health system, bringing health care as close as possible to where people live and work.③ Primary care constitutes the first element of a continuing health care process that may also include the provision of timely and appropriate secondary and tertiary levels of care, but it is important to note that the IOM suggests timing could lead to strict conceptualizations. Therefore, the IOM states that "chief, principal or main" are preferred descriptors.

3.1.2.3 Health

PHC is rooted in contemporary conceptualizations of health as a biopsychosocial phenomenon and not simply the absence of disease. A PHC orientation to health services delivery recognizes individual, family, community and population experiences of health and illness, as well as the ways in which health and health care are situated within specific social, historical and political contexts. The experiences of marginalized peoples have contributed to more robust conceptualizations of health. Thus, efforts to improve health should draw upon the knowledge of each of the health professions, as well as knowledge situated in cognate disciplines and the various other stakeholders in health care, thereby creating a dynamic dialogue that is reflective of the vitality of interdisciplinary efforts.

---

① Tarlier D S, Johnson J L, Whyte N B. Voices from the Wilderness: An Interpretive Study Describing the Role and Practice of Outpost Nurses [J]. Canadian Journal of Public Health/Revue Canadienne de Sante'e Publique, 2003: 180-184.

② Institute of Medicine (US). Division of Health Care Services. Committee on the Future of Primary Care. Donaldson M S, Vanselow N A, et al. Defining Primary Care: An Interim Report. National Academy Press, 1994.

③ Stevenson R M, Hogg W, Huston P. Integrating Public Health and Primary Care[J]. Healthc Policy, 2007, 3: e160-e181.

PHC forms an integral part of the country's health system. While the main focus of PHC is the health of individuals, families, and communities, PHC is equally concerned with addressing the overall social and economic development of communities, thereby targeting the social determinants of health. PHC embodies a spirit of self-reliance and self-determination①; it is driven by and suggests community empowerment and building community capacity and resilience, "the fundamental premise of community development is that when people are given the opportunity to work out their own problems, they will find solutions that will have a more lasting effect than when they are not involved in such problem solving"②. Therefore, PHC implies essential community-based health care that (1) is generally accessible to individuals, families, groups, communities and populations; (2) is driven by community participation in identifying health issues; (3) involves community participation in decision-making regarding appropriate solutions; (4) is sustainable by the community.

The philosophical underpinnings of PHC direct attention to both the art and science of patient-centered primary care, while recognizing that the relationship between health and health care is not always reflective of a linear progression through various stages of illness and treatment. Working within a PHC model, primary care provider roles are differentiated from conventional medical model provider roles by the "notion of working with rather than caring for"③, implying a shift in thinking that WHO described as giving professional health workers "a new orientation". A PHC orientation to the provision of primary care recognizes the value of "looking upstream", "seeing the bigger picture", and "realizing that band aid solutions don't work, we need to get to the root of the problems"④. In practice, a PHC orientation can provide new challenges and opportunities for teaching, as well as research⑤.

3.2   The Subject of Primary Health Care

The subject of PHC and the role of the PHC provider have recently been gradually valued. There may be general understanding of the term—primary health care, but its exact meaning has

---

① Vukic A, Keddy B. Northern Nursing Practice in a Primary Health Care Setting [J]. Journal of Advanced Nursing, 2002, 40(5): 542-548.

② Lindsey E, Sheilds L, Stajduhar K. Creating Effective Nursing Partnerships: Relating Community Development to Participatory Action Research[J]. Journal of Advanced Nursing, 1999, 29(5): 1238-1245.

③ Palmer C N A, Ismail T, Lee S P, et al. Filaggrin Null Mutations are Associated with Increased Asthma Severity in Children and Young Adults[J]. Journal of Allergy and Clinical Immunology, 2007, 120(1): 64-68.

④ Tarlier D S, Johnson J L, Whyte N B. Voices from the Wilderness: An Interpretive Study Describing the Role and Practice of Outpost Nurses [J]. Canadian Journal of Public Health/Revue Canadienne de Sante'e Publique, 2003: 180-184.

⑤ Schultz W. Predictive Reward Signal of Dopamine Neurons[J]. Journal of Neurophysiology, 1998, 80(1): 1-27.

been improperly described, thus making it difficult to define its content and the scope of the role of the primary health care provider. Many take PHC only as initial care, the care resulting from first contact. Others consider it as dealing mainly with the acute medical aspects of health care and, in particular, those aspects having to do with illness and disease. Still others relate PHC to "family medicine", "ambulatory medicine", "personal medicine", or "nonspecialist care".

PHC is more than any or all of these. The term is not suitable for a specific or brief definition, but requires a relatively lengthy description to give a full picture of its content and scope since it involves a broad range of care and services that are central and essential to the health and well-beings of individuals and families.

PHC includes the initial contact of the patient with the health care system, and provides high-quality, individualized, comprehensive, quickly responsive, and readily accessible care. It is also patient-oriented, easy to use, and based on a firm foundation which integrates multidisciplinary knowledge, namely medicine, biology, social psychology, and behavioral sciences.

3.2.1   The Functions of Primary Health Care

The basic functions of primary health care include the followings:

(1) The care of the well and the sick seen principally in ambulatory settings.

(2) The provision of a full range of basic health services.

(3) The continuing care and management of the chronically ill, the disabled, and those requiring recovery.

(4) The diagnosis and therapy of a wide variety of illnesses and injuries including the screening, initial care, management, and triage of surgical and medical emergencies.

(5) The responsibility for recognizing and evaluating patients' total health needs, particularly those that are serious and correctable.

(6) The provision of psychological and emotional support to help people deal with psychosocial problems and psychosomatic responses, to live with stress, and be relieved of some anxiety.

(7) The promotion of health through genetic counseling, family planning, sex education, nutritional counseling, and other forms of counseling and health education.

(8) The assessment and management of individuals with learning and retention difficulties, memory defects, and perceptual problems.

(9) The prevention of infectious disease, trauma, and disorders secondary to environmental hazards.

(10) The provision to the individual of health advice and services to promote health maintenance at an optimal level and to increase patients' capabilities to assume responsibility for their own care.

(11) The identification of individuals at special risk from various congenital and acquired

disorders.

(12) The referral of the patient, when necessary, to appropriate resources, specialists, and others, and the guidance of the patient through various levels of health care.

3.2.2 Connotations of Primary Health Care

PHC may have different connotations for different groups, each of whom may emphasize specific components and implications of particular interest or importance to them, but may disregard the full scope and meaning of the term.

For the government, the emphasis on the training of health professionals to be primary health care providers is a means of achieving improved distribution of health care providers, particularly in rural areas, and to counteract the overemphasis that some believed has been placed in recent years on research. The government and others need a descriptive definition of PHC so they can have a clearer understanding of its scope and content, and can develop more realistic and significant legislation that will include achievable goals.

For the specialties of pediatrics, internal medicine, obstetrics and gynecology, and psychiatry, PHC is a designation that they now seek to have more strongly applied to their disciplines so that their training programs may become eligible for funding when financial supports from the federal government and other sources become available for the training of PHC providers. Medical specialties need a comprehensively descriptive definition to serve as the basis in determining the content of training programs. When they get a better understanding of the content and scope of PHC relating to their disciplines, they can realize the importance of PHC in their specialties and be in a position to make the experience they provide their trainees more pertinent and effective in preparing them as health care providers.

To the public, the term PHC is an unfamiliar one. In general, the public is more concerned with the accessibility of PHC than its exact content or the capability of the PHC providers to serve as a highly competent health professional with sufficient knowledge to provide the varied services. A better understanding of the scope and content of PHC provides consumers with the knowledge they need to know what to expect from PHC providers and to be in a position to judge the adequacy of the care they receive.

For educational institutions, particularly those receiving financial supports from state legislatures, PHC is seen as the "bandwagon" on which they had better climb since it may be the only way for them to stay solvent now that research support and private donations have decreased. Although educational institutions recognize the importance of increasing their investment in the area of PHC, they may not be entirely clear as to the place that PHC should have in their curricula and overall operations; they may not have decided how to expand the teaching of PHC in an already overcrowded schedule; and they may be uncertain as to what to cover, who needs to be prepared to do what, or how to get their graduates to go where they are needed. PHC represents the area of the curriculum in many medical schools that has been largely neglected in the past; it assumes strikingly increased importance when educators realize that many of the influential legislators who control medical school budgets are elected from rural areas and that these legislators see PHC as the way to fill the unmet health needs of their constituents. Educational institutions need a comprehensive descriptive definition of PHC, so they will know what curriculum modifications are required to prepare more qualified PHC providers to meet the health needs of the public.

For nurses, PHC can serve as the key to an expanded role in the health care system and the means by which service-oriented nurses such as nurse practitioners who practice as providers of direct PHC can achieve improved status and a more competitive position vis-a-vis administrative "higher degree" nurses in obtaining the recognition (and income) they deserve for their clinical abilities and professional contributions. Nursing needs an acceptable descriptive definition of PHC, so it can further adapt and expand the educational experience which its students and graduates receive in PHC and better prepare them to meet a greater portion of the total health care needs of the public.

The comprehensive definition of PHC described delineates its scope and content, allows health professionals and the public to communicate more effectively regarding it, serves as the basis in determining the content of training programs required to prepare PHC providers, more adequately describes the potential role of health care providers, and increases consumers' knowledge, so they can know what to expect from PHC providers and can be in a position to judge the adequacy of the care they receive.

3.3   Management for Primary Health Care

If primary health care services are to improve, so must management services. The critical aspects of the role of a PHC manager and some of the skills necessary to carry out for this role, are outlined. The concept of PHC management is compared and contrasted with other forms of management.

It will become clear throughout the discussion that PHC management is shared management, not only between the employees of the organization, but also with the community they serve. Indeed, this partnership with the community is one of the major notions that separates PHC management from other forms of management. In practice, it demands a great deal of managerial skill to establish and negotiate continually shared values and yet present an organizational exterior to the world which says: "We believe in what we are doing, we know where we are going, and we want to form a cooperative partnership with you in order to get there." Because of the strong community support system fundamental to PHC, it is often the case that a health service based on the principles of PHC might from time to time look as if it lacks direction. This can happen when the service is actually being a service and is actively seeking community direction, rather than planning and making the decisions itself. The skills needed for a PHC manager to deal with key players outside the organization are as important, if not more so, than those needed to facilitate internal management①.

3.3.1　Primary Health Care Management Differs from Traditional Health Care Management

PHC is "health for the people by the people", and seeks to address deficiencies in empowerment, collaboration in health, community control over health and lives, equality, justice, self-reliance, and self-determination.

Management means a group of activities that need to be performed to some degree by all individuals within the organization in order for the organization to achieve its mission. It is not the exclusive domain of those who occupy the highest levels on the organizational chart, those who earn the most money, or those who think they have the answers. It is a shared activity for all team members and the team must include members of the community, for it is the community that defines the mission of the organization and its modus operandi.

Many health systems claim to have a community participation component, although often this is limited to recommendations being made at meetings, in community surveys and so on. This might be termed "community involvement", but it is not "participation" which means to take part in.

In practice, this means that a PHC service continually takes its direction from the people whose health the service hopes to affect. The role of management in PHC then is to convert community ideas into practice. The community reflects on these actions and gives the service new direction. This is one of many PHC spirals and cycles, as PHC is always evolving, always dynamic.

PHC management knows no monopolies. One person might be designated manager or coordinator and be paid accordingly but still share the functions of management in such a way that all team members, employees and community are empowered. The type of management necessary for this approach to health care will necessarily be different from the management that worked in the traditional top down: "medical model" of health care. The implementation of PHC is about changing the power structure in health care (Figure 3-1).②③④

The structure of power within PHC management is flattered, management is shared, and autonomy and collaboration are primary as part of the culture: The adoption of a broad span of

---

①　Johnson S. Management for Primary Health Care[J]. Australian Journal of Primary Health, 1996.

②　Werner D, Bower B. Helping Health Workers Learn[J]. Studies in Family Planning, 1984, 15(2).

③　Johnson S. Aboriginal health through primary health care[J]. G., Gray, R. Pratt, (Eds.), Issues in Australian Nursing, 1992, 3: 151-170.

④　Rifkin S B. Health planning and community participation: case studies in South-East Asia[M]. Taylor & Francis, 1985.

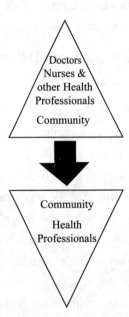

Figure 3-1   Power Structure in Primary Health Care
(Source: Johnson S. Management for Primary Health Care[J].
Australian Journal of Primary Health, 1996.)

control makes it impossible for any line manager to control others too tightly. The end result is that managers lose their sense of learned helplessness and dependency on others and learn to act for themselves①. The role of the assigned manager in this type of structure is crucial, since the manager should make sure that in this circumstance of collaboration roles are not blurred, responsibility is not avoided, and authority is maintained. In the initial stages of implementation, care must be taken through the provision of clear direction to avoid destruction to services.

The skills of the designated manager and the team vary little from those described under new business management styles, such as "new organizational theory"②. It is this type of statement that reveals "new management theory" as being close to PHC management. Consistent with the principles of PHC, managers of health systems must model a "people-centered" approach. Their style, however, although not necessarily different from new mainstream business management, will differ considerably from the management practices prevalent in

---

①   Limerick D, Cunnington B. Managing the New Organization: A Blueprint for Networks and Strategic Alliances[M]. Chatwood, NSW: Business & Professional Publishing,1993.

②   National Aboriginal Health Strategy Working Party (Australia). A National Aboriginal Health Strategy [M]. Canberra: National Aboriginal Health Strategy Working Party, 1989.

traditional mainstream hierarchical organizations. Although it is still important to "get the job done", PHC focuses more on "how" the job is done, and on how the process ensures empowerment and collaboration.

For the indigenous people of Australia, health "refers to the social, emotional and cultural well-being of the whole community"①. Those of us who have been privileged to work beside Aboriginal people would have seen this system in action and it is hoped would have realized how much our society could learn from it if prepared to listen. It is no accident that the first network of PHC services in Australia (begun in 1971), had been built against great odds by the indigenous people. The main idea for this network, is reflexed in current writings about business management: The central idea of the new organization is that of emancipated, autonomous, empowered individuals managing their own collaboration towards a shared purpose②.

The conclusions drawn in this article flow from an experience where different types of management were tried and many mistakes made, until it was clear that only one type of management worked for the particular PHC service. The following is an overview of that experience and practical examples will be drawn to clarify particular points.

The role and style of the manager is crucial in the dynamic spiral of change of PHC and, as illustrated above, it leaves the manager in an extremely vulnerable position. Best practice in PHC management is not about being comfortable and secure, however, the continual challenge makes one "feel activated".

3.3.2 Critical Skills of a PHC Manager

Best practice for a PHC manager demands many and varied skills, but perhaps the most important of these, which differ from the skills required of a more traditional health manager, lie in the area of enabling, of facilitating; these catalytic skills and others will allow the manager to be effective③:

(1) Negotiate shared management;

(2) Build receptivity to change;

(3) Facilitate the circumstance for empowerment;

(4) Model negotiation;

(5) Act as a cultural broker;

(6) Perform the functions of a cultural safety officer;

---

① National Aboriginal Health Strategy Working Party (Australia). A National Aboriginal Health Strategy [M]. Canberra: National Aboriginal Health Strategy Working Party, 1989.

② National Aboriginal Health Strategy Working Party (Australia). A National Aboriginal Health Strategy [M]. Canberra: National Aboriginal Health Strategy Working Party, 1989.

③ Johnson S. Management for Primary Health Care [J]. Australian Journal of Primary Health, 1996.

(7) Play a role as a buffer for "accountability stress";

(8) Create and maintain strategic alliances.

3.3.3   Some Suggestions about Management ①

3.3.3.1   Negotiating Shared Management

The skills required of the manager are in reality no different from the management skills required by all members of the team. However, the difference between them is the emphasis that the manager should press on the use of extraordinary skills at particular times and the processes that bring these changes about. The assigned manager needs to be most skilled at forecasting and detecting change within a dynamic organization. Ideally, as members of the team become more skilled, the assigned manager will negotiate his (or her) role again, placing less and less emphasis on the areas covered by the team members' newly developed skill areas, and more in the areas newly identified through negotiation, as in need of attention. This is one of the rewarding aspects of management for PHC as the role constantly changes and exposes diverse challenges.

3.3.3.2   Building Receptivity to Change

Because PHC is still new to public, one of the primary tasks for a PHC manager is to prepare the organization for change, this includes building awareness, understanding and commitment to the implementation of PHC. The success of the task depends on managers, nevertheless, for the purpose of being effective, they need to have a clear mandate for this from the organization.

As well as preparing the organization for change, the PHC manager also has a responsibility to promote consciousness within the community about the changed role of individuals within the health service. People who have been oppressed often prefer to have a health service that tells them what to do.

3.3.3.3   Acting as a Cultural Broker

Someone points out that the business press, starting sometime in 1980, has increasingly used culture as a metaphor of its own, it is often referred to as corporate culture. "The leader is the creator of symbols, ideologies, language, beliefs, rituals, and myths"②. Set against this

---

① Johnson S. Management for Primary Health Care[J]. Australian Journal of Primary Health, 1996.

② Peter T J, Waterman R H. In search of excellence: Lessons from America's best-run companies[J]. New York: Warner Book, 1984.

definition of corporate culture, is the conception of PHC management as shared management① :

(1) A blueprint for all human behavior;

(2) The communication of meaning;

(3) A view of the world that has meaning;

(4) The interactions of human beings in terms of symbols with shared meanings.

Just as community participation is the "lifeblood of the philosophy" of PHC, so negotiation of shared meaning is the organizational culture's 'lifeblood'. It is through this "communication of meaning" that the PHC organization's view of the world is established as a "blueprint" for organizational behavior. In this context then the role of the manager is to promote the shaping of shared meaning: "The management of collaboration is, in the end, the management of identity and meaning."②. Beyond the notion of the manager as the promoter of the organizational culture and its linked symbols, is the far more powerful concept of cultural safety.

3.3.3.4 Being a Cultural Safety Officer

In suiting these conceptions to PHC management, best practice requires that one of the major skills requirment of a manager is to guarantee the cultural safety of an organization, not only by facilitating the frequent renegotiation of its shared values in view of its own development and ever changing environment, but also by making the PHC structures visible to those external to the organization. This is necessary because the basic functions of management, for example planning, staffing, organizing, controlling and leading, are all undertaken to varying degrees by all team members. One of the results of these shared management roles is that PHC organizations "look" very different from other more conventional systems of management. More conventional organizations have well entrenched notions of interacting and are usually confused by this new look, which is threatening to the comfortable status quo. So there is a tendency to misunderstand the new system and to value it less than the more conventional organization with which most people are familiar.

Another aspect of cultural safety for PHC, is that it is important for political commitment to the implementation of PHC. If the government bureaucracy is target or outcome driven, then for short term goals the PHC process might seem inefficient.

3.3.3.5 Creating and Maintaining Strategic Alliances

The networks that a manager of PHC must make and maintain are both internal and

---

① Eckermann A K, Dowd T, Chong E, et al. Binan Goonj: bridging cultures in Aboriginal health[M]. NSW: University of New England Press, 1992.

② Limerick D, Cunnington B. Managing the New organization: A Blueprint for Networks and Strategic Alliances[M]. Chatwood, NSW: Business & Professional Publishing, 1993.

external to the organization. The internal network is an empowering, collaborative system which includes the community and is grounded on the twin themes of autonomy and interdependence. The skill of the manager is the most important in balancing the twin perceptions of cultural safety and empowered interdependence.

Against the background of the holistic nature of PHC, political lobbying is a narrow concept which presupposes an existing imbalance of power. The PHC organization, which is relatively small, when interacting with a major power like the government, is disadvantaged. Negotiation cannot occur unless each player comes to the table feeling an equal level of power. A more productive partnership can be developed between the organization and the wider community of which is a part (e.g., government, bureaucracy, media) through the developing of strategic alliances; in part this depends on the organization strengthening its culture and declaring its space.

3.3.4   Conclusion

One of the reasons why best practice in PHC management different from the traditional health system management is because of the strong community participation in PHC. It promotes health care towards a more "people-centered" way.

PHC also drives the construction of the health system towards a more collaborative one where management is transparent (not vague). There is greater interdependence without losing autonomy both inside and outside the organization.

Strategic alliances, especially outside the organization, are a healthier way to deal with political questions than to continue down the disempowering track of accepting lesser status because the PHC organization is more "grassroots", or smaller, or composed mainly of women. Real negotiation can come into being through strategic alliances where people are equal.

Management for PHC can be summarized as a shared management of identity and meaning. An organization where shared meanings are frequently renegotiated is a powerful organization. Its staff will feel more willing to give full play to their ability and work collaboration with each other towards a shared purpose, this results in empowerment and purpose being achieved. Valid cooperative management is significant for the successful implementation and advancing maintenance of best practice in PHC[1].

---

[1]   Johnson S. Management for Primary Health Care[J]. Australian Journal of Primary Health, 1996.

Chapter 4   Introduction to Public Health Administration

Public health is the foundation of a healthy society. To understand and improve public health require that one do more than aggregate what one understands about individual health. We know some of the components that influence individual health: genetic predisposition or determination, social background, disposable income, climate, advances in health technologies and caring protocols, organizational capacity for multi-sectoral and multidisciplinary working, peer influence, personality, motivation, capacity and willingness to look after oneself and one's family, friends and neighbors. There is great diversity and abundance of subjects that concern public health professionals. Typically, public health professionals discuss the following topics:

(1) Dating and Intimate Partner Violence;

(2) Promoting Post-disaster Resilience and Mental Health Through Community Capacity Building in New Orleans;

(3) Creating Community Advocates Using a Critical Health Literacy Model;

(4) Portable Farmer's Market: Mobile Vending to Promote Healthy Food Access in Vulnerable Communities;

(5) An Initiative to Apply Health Protection Mechanisms in International Trade Regulations;

(6) Digital Disparities: The Role of Technology/HIT in the Development and Elimination of Health Disparities;

(7) Health Care Reform.

Furthermore, there is a variety of answers responding to "what is public health?" The answers may be as following:

(1) When I think of public health, I think of early intervention, prevention.

(2) Public health is immunization, school health, control of contagious disease.

(3) It's anything that affects the health of the community on a mass basis.

(4) Public health is the area of health outside the capability of the individual private practitioner.

(5) The core of public health is the capacity to identify problems, and find them, measure them and attempt to intervene.

However, public health system is the cornerstone for the population in countries across the world. For public health, one needs to know what public health means to individuals within a society or population and consider the context in which individuals and societies live. One needs to know the fundamental theories and models that underlying in public health programs, and how governmental sectors run the public system and fulfill their functions in the system. One also needs to know how to evaluate the system and lead different departments, organizations, social groups to work together to cope with the major public health issues efficiently and effectively. Yet these are this chapter intends to do.

4.1　Overview of Public Health

4.1.1　Definition of Public Health

As a society we seem to assume that we are fully capable of maintaining past progress (often dramatic improvements in the public health and longevity), of addressing current problems, and of being prepared to respond to new crises or emergent health problems. The broad mission of public health is to "fulfill society's interest in assuring conditions in which people can be healthy". (IOM, 1988) According to this statement, Public health is what we, as a society, do collectively to assure the conditions for people to be healthy. By this definition, we understand public practices' commonalities with other practices focused on health— particularly the clinical practices such as medicine, nursing, dentistry, physical therapy, and others—as well as the unique role of public health.

Firstly, the idea of assuring health for all people—the entire population—is embedded in the mission and definition of public health. Although public health will focus on different populations within the larger population when planning services, we are obligated to ensure health-producing conditions for all people— not just the poor, not just the rich, but people of all incomes; not only the young or the old, but people of all ages; not exclusively Whites or Blacks, but people of all races and ethnicities.

Secondly, the belief that a society benefit from having a healthy populace is clear in the public health mission's phrase "to fulfill society's interest ..." The work of public health is a societal effort with a societal benefit. Public health takes the view held by many professions and societies throughout human history that healthy people are more productive and creative, and these attributes create a strong society. Healthy people lead to better societies. For the welfare of the society, as a whole, it is better for people to be healthy than sick. There will be less dependence, less lost time from productive work, and a greater pool of productive workers, soldiers, parents, and others needed to accomplish society's goals. Thus, as public health professionals, we believe that society has an interest in the health of the population; it benefits the society, as a whole, when people are healthy.

Thirdly, the public health mission acknowledges that health is not guaranteed. The mission states that "people can/will(not) be healthy". Health is a possibility, although we intend to make it highly probable through our actions. However, not everyone will be healthy even if each one exists in health-producing conditions. Public health efforts will not result in every person being healthy—although we certainly would not object to that kind of success. Rather, public health creates conditions in which people can be healthy. Whether any single individual is healthy, we acknowledge, will vary.

4.1.2 Practices of Public Health

If we examine the definition of public health closely, we find that public health is complementary to the clinical practices, but not subsumed by it. The critical differences between public health and the clinical practices relate to their strategies for creating a healthy populace. Prevention is the preferred strategy and to be successful, prevention must address the conditions, in which people live. The classic and defining public health strategy is to prevent poor health by "assuring conditions in which people can be healthy".

4.1.2.1 Definition of Prevention

There are three types of prevention: primary, secondary, and tertiary. Fos and Fine (2000) define primary, secondary, and tertiary prevention as follows:

Primary prevention is concerned with eliminating risk factors for a disease. Secondary prevention focuses on early detection and treatment of disease (subclinical and clinical). Tertiary prevention attempts to eliminate or moderate disability associated with advanced disease.

Primary prevention intends to prevent the development of disease and the occurrence of injury, and, to reduce their incidence in the population. Examples of primary prevention include the use of automobile seat belts, condom use, skin protection from ultraviolet light, and tobacco-use cessation programs. Secondary prevention is concerned with treating disease after it has developed so that there are no permanent adverse consequences; early detection is emphasized. Secondary prevention activities are intended to identify the existence of disease early so that treatments that might not be as effective when applied later can be of benefit. Tertiary prevention focuses on the optimum treatment of clinically apparent and clearly identified disease to reduce complications to the greatest possible degree. Tertiary prevention usually refers to reduce disability caused by disease and injury being not treated effectively.

4.1.2.2 Determinants of Health

What is entailed in "assuring conditions in which people can be healthy"? The answer to this question lies the source of the varied interests, knowledge, and skills that differentiate public health practice from each other. The causes of poor health are many and complex, and therefore, solutions are complex and diverse, as well. Before we discuss the theoretical models tackling this complexity in public health practices, we will discuss how we define health and conceptualize the complex set of factors that affect health, called the determinants of health.

In the 1940s, the World Health Organization (WHO) stated that "Health is a state of complete physical, mental and social wellbeing and not merely, the absence of disease or infirmity". However, the WHO definition is "honored in repetition, rarely in application". In general public health practice, the term health will refer to the more restricted definition— diagnosable morbidity, disability, and premature mortality.

With either broad definition of health, or more narrow perspective, there are many influences on individual and population health. It is generally accepted that the determinants of health include the physical environment—natural and built—and the social environment, as well as individual behavior, genetic inheritance, and health care (Evans & Stoddart, 1994). Note that although we talk about the "determinants of health", they are usually discussed in terms of how they relate to poor health—the determinants of poor health. A brief overview of the determinants of health follows.

Physical environment includes both the natural and the built environments. The natural environment is defined by the features of an area that include its topography, weather, soil, water, animal life, and other such attributes; and the built environment is defined by the structures that people have created for housing, commerce, transportation, government, recreation, and so forth. Health threats arise from both the natural and the built environments. Common health threats related to the natural environment include weather-related disasters such as tornados, hurricanes, and earthquakes, as well as exposure to infectious disease agents that are endemic in a region. Health threats related to the built environment include exposure to toxins and unsafe conditions, particularly in occupational and residential settings where people spend most of their time.

The social environment is defined by the major organizing concepts of human life: society, community, religion, social network, family, and occupation. Individuals' lives are governed by religious, political, economic, and organizational rules—formal and informal—that reflect the cultural norms, values, and beliefs of their particular social context. These formal and informal rules, an important aspect of the social environment is the status, resources, and power that individuals have within their social environment or context and the values, beliefs and norms they reflect, have historical roots, and they affect how individuals live and behave; their relationships with others; and what resources and opportunities individuals have to influence their lives. They shape the relationship between individuals and the natural environment and how the built environment is conceived and developed.

Genetic inheritance on health is well accepted and recognized by both public health professionals and clinicians as well. It is understood that, with few exceptions, disease processes "are determined both by environmental and by genetic factors. These usually interact, and individuals with a particular set of genes may be either more or less likely, if exposed, to be at risk of developing a particular disease. These effects can be measured by showing that the relative risk of exposure to an environmental factor is significantly greater (or lesser) for the subgroup with the abnormal gene, than the risk in those without" (Pencheon, Guest, Melzer, & Gray, 2001).

Health behavior can refer to behaviors that are beneficial to health. However, the term is generally used in the negative to refer to behaviors that harm health, including smoking, abusing alcohol or other substances, failing to use seat belts or practicing other unsafe behaviors, making unhealthy food choices, and not engaging in adequate physical activity. The effect of health behaviors on health status has been widely studied and found to be an important determinant of health. In one way or another, personal health behavior has an impact on the occurrence in any given individual of most of the diseases and conditions on the list of leading causes of death in both industrial countries and most developing countries as well.

If we argue that health is the product of multiple factors including genetic inheritance, the physical environment, and the social environment, as well as an individual's behavioral and biologic response to these factors, we see that health care has an impact on the causal chain leading to disease, illness, and injury. Often by the time the individual interacts with the health care system, the determinants of health have had their impact on their health status, for better or for worse. Thus, the need for health care may be seen as a failure to prevent the determinants of health from adversely affecting the individual patient.

4.1.2.3 Priorities and Essential Services in Public Health

According to what we discussed so far, for public health practices, it is needed to do more than quantify the sum, or the mean, of the health of all the individuals within a society and consider the context in which individuals and societies live. Within this mission fall a number of characteristic themes, which over the course of a long historical tradition have coalesced around the goal of the people's health. Early public health focused on sanitary measures and the control of communicable disease. With the discovery of bacteria and immunologic advances, disease prevention was added to the subject matter of public health. (Hanlon and Pickett, 1984) In recent decades, health promotion has become an increasingly important theme, as the interrelationship among the physical, mental, and social dimensions of well-being has been clarified. Over time, the substance of public health has expanded. With its inherent complexity, public health practices need to set priorities with the limited resources. Governmental sectors or agencies play critical roles in setting the goals and guiding the practices. 10 public health objectives in Sweden are as follows:

(1) Participation and influence in society;
(2) Economic and social security;
(3) Secure and favorable conditions during childhood and adolescence;
(4) Healthier working life;
(5) Healthy and safe environments and products;

（6）Health and medical care that more actively promotes good health；

（7）Effective protection against communicable diseases；

（8）Safe sexuality and good reproductive health；

（9）Increased physical activity；

（10）Good eating habits and safe food.

National public health objectives reflect the configuration of the priorities in the public health strategies in one country. However, these objectives are strategic. Public practices need to identify the daily or routine activities or services to make up the gap between system practices and system strategies. The following 10 essential public health services were identified by the Center for Disease Control and Prevention in the United States：

（1）Monitor health status to identify community health problems；

（2）Diagnose and investigate health problems and health hazards in the community；

（3）Inform, educate, and empower people on health issues；

（4）Mobilize community partnerships to identify and solve health problems；

（5）Develop policies and plans that support individual and community health efforts；

（6）Enforce laws and regulations that protect health and ensure safety；

（7）Link people to needed personal health services and assure the provision of health care when otherwise unavailable；

（8）Assure a competent public health and personal health care workforce；

（9）Evaluate effectiveness, accessibility, and quality of personal and population-based health services；

（10）Research for new insights and innovative solutions to health problems.

4.1.3   Theoretical Models of Public Health Practices

4.1.3.1   Ecological Models

The environment, or context, influences the way people live and their health outcomes, for better or for worse. That is context can have positive or negative impacts on the health of individuals. The way in which public health attempts to affect contexts is the story of public health practice, and public health practice reflects public health ecological models. However, the ecological models in use change over time to respond to the health problems predominant in their day and incorporate the knowledge, beliefs, values, and resources of that time and place.

For example, in times and places where infectious diseases are predominant, models reflect the issues required to understand their spread and control. A classic public health model that uses the ecological approach for understanding and preventing disease is the epidemiological triangle with its agent-host-environment triad. The epidemiological triangle （see Figure 4-1）was developed and is used to understand infectious disease transmission and to provide a model for preventing transmission, and thus, infectious disease outbreaks. The three points of the triangle are the agent, host, and environment. The agent is the microbial organism that causes the infectious disease—virus, bacteria, protozoa, or fungus; the host is the organism that harbors the agent; and the environmental aspects included in an epidemiological triangle are those factors that facilitate transmission of the agent to the host. These could be aspects of the natural environment, the built environment, or the social environment, including policies. Time is considered in the triangle as the period between exposure to the agent and illness occurs; the period that it takes to recover from illness; or the period it takes an outbreak to subside. Prevention measures are those that disrupt the relationship between at least two of the factors in the triangle—agent, host, and environment.

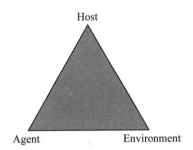

Figure 4-1 Epidemiological Triangle

The wheel of causation is another model exemplifying the ecological approach (See Figure 4-2). It has also been used, but not as extensively as the epidemiological triangle for explaining infectious disease transmission. However, it has some advantages over the epidemiological triangle, as Peterson (1995) notes. Although it is not used as often as the epidemiological triangle model, it has several appealing attributes. For instance, the wheel contains a hub with the host at its center. For our use, humans represent the host. Also, surrounding the host is the total environment divided into the biological, physical, and social environments. These divisions, of course, are not true divisions—there are considerable interactions among the environment types. Although it is a general model, the wheel of causation does illustrate the multiple etiological factors of human infectious diseases.

In general, every ecological model explaining the development of health (or poor health) contains a set of distal causes related to the environment—physical and/or social—and a set of proximal causes related to the individual—primarily behavioral. One of the major issues in developing public health models is where to place the emphasis and, thus, where to intervene to improve health? Is it at the individual level or at the environmental level? This issue is at the heart of public health practice.

4.1.3.2 Health Promotion Models

Beginning in the 1960s, the models explaining health status became increasingly limited to

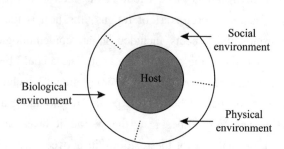

Figure 4-2   Wheel of Causation

the behavioral determinants of health such as smoking, sedentary lifestyle, poor dietary habits, unprotected sexual activity, and failure to use seat belts, which placed the focus of public health interventions on changing individuals rather than their context. The watchwords of this trend were health promotion and disease prevention. As Green (1999) stated, 1974 was a turning point when health promotion was accepted as a significant component of health policy. In a classic review of the rise in importance of health promotion, McLeroy, Bibeau, Steckler, and Glanz (1988) summarized the events and initiatives characterizing the ascendance during the 1970s and 1980s. The emphasis on health promotion, however, increasingly emphasized public health initiatives at the individual behavior level, rather than the environmental level. Programs to help people stop smoking, lose weight, increase exercise, eat healthier foods, and so forth proliferated, and these programs were predominantly aimed at educating and motivating individuals to change unhealthy behaviors. These initiatives were in contrast to historic interventions such as sewage disposal or food inspection that emphasized changing the environment.

Most health promotion programs used the now well-known model for conceptualizing community health promotion and planning: Green and Kreuter's (1991, 1999) PRECEDE-PROCEED model. The PRECEDE-PROCEED model was developed in the 1970s and has been applied, since then with a few modifications in the 1990s, which we will discuss shortly. PRECEDE stands for Predisposing, Reinforcing, and Enabling Construction Educational Diagnosis and Evaluation. PROCEED stands for Policy, Regulatory, and Organizational Constructs in Educational and Environmental Development. Predisposing factors are defined as a person's or population's knowledge, attitudes, beliefs, values, and perceptions that facilitate or hinder motivation for change. Enabling factors are those skills, resources, or barriers that can help or hinder the desired behavioral changes as well as environmental changes. Reinforcing factors, the rewards received, and the feedback the learner receives from others following adoption of the behavior, may encourage or discourage continuation of the behavior.

The model is oriented toward improving health by changing individuals' behavior through education, and not toward intervening at the environmental level to change conditions or structures. The question structured by PRECEDE-PROCEED model is "Why do people behave badly, that is, engaging in unhealthy behaviors?" In addition, the first part of the two-part answer to this question, which is emphasized by PRECEDE-PROCEED, is lack of knowledge.

Thus, education about the risks of certain behaviors and the benefits of others is a primary component of health promotion initiatives. These include initiatives to modify unfavorable dietary habits, sedentary lifestyle, substance abuse, smoking, and unsafe practices such as failure to use seat belts or follow safety precautions at work. The second part of the answer structured by this model is related to attributes of the individual that hinder behavior change including motivation to change, appraisal of threat, self-efficacy, response efficacy, and so forth. That is, once the knowledge about health behaviors is conveyed, the challenge is to motivate individuals to change their behavior from risky to healthy. Knowledge alone is not sufficient to bring about change in health behaviors. Thus, a major tool of health promotion is the application of psychological theories to understand why people engage in unhealthy behaviors and how to stimulate them to modify these behaviors.

The PRECEDE-PROCEED model (See Figure 4-3) visualizes the assumed causal chain, which shows that behavioral problems produce health problems, which then in turn, produce social problems, such as illegitimacy, unemployment, absenteeism, hostility, alienation,

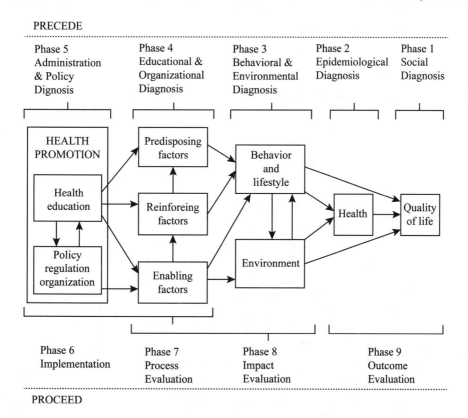

Figure 4-3　The PRECEDE-PROCEED Model for Health Promotion Planning and Evaluation

discrimination, riots, and crime. The effect of the environment on individual behavior is assumed under enabling factors such as availability of resources, accessibility, and referrals and reinforcing factors as attitudes of program personnel. However, note that this is a very restricted environment, which is limited to the immediate setting of the health education program. There is also a non-behavioral factors box, which contributes to health problems and could contain larger environmental factors, but is not the main focus of the model and is not seen as contributing to behavior problems.

4.1.3.3 Health Impact Pyramid

The health impact pyramid developed by Frieden (2010) provides a very useful framework for integrating the ecological and health promotion models into public health practice (see Figure 4-4). "A 5-tier pyramid best describes the impact of different types of public health interventions and provides a framework to improve health. At the base of this pyramid, indicating interventions with the greatest potential impact, are efforts to address socio-economic determinants of health. In ascending order are interventions that change the context to make individuals' default decisions healthy, clinical interventions that require limited contact but confer long-term protection, and ongoing directly clinical care, and health education and counseling" (Frieden, 2010). Note that the author accepts the population health perspective that structural inequality embodied in socioeconomic factors is the level with the most potential to improve health—a primary prevention strategy. Also note that the second level—changing the context—is a primary prevention strategy, which includes provision of clean water and safe food, as well as passage of laws that prevent injuries and exposure to disease-producing agents.

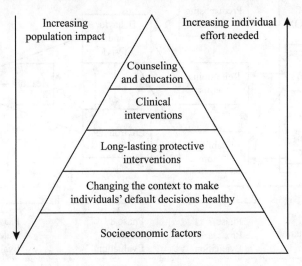

Figure 4-4 The Health Impact Pyramid

Interventions at the top tiers are a mix of primary, secondary, and tertiary prevention "designed to help individuals, rather than entire populations, but they could theoretically have a large population impact if universally and effectively applied. In practice, however, even the best programs at the pyramid's higher levels achieve limited public health impact, largely because of their dependence on long-term individual behavior change".

4.2 Organization and Financing of Public Health

4.2.1 Conceptual Elements of Public Health

From the beginning of our discussion, we believe that it is important not to limit understanding of "public health" to what health departments do. Instead, it aims to place government activities within a broader framework that can guide a wide range of institutional participants. The intent is not to emphasize the role of the public agency. On the contrary, it is to point out the indispensability of its prerogatives and functions by calling attention to the context in which they are exercised. This distinction between "public health" and "what health departments do" is implicated in the definition of public health proposed by Institute of Medicine in the United States. The definition has three parts: (1) the mission of public health: a statement of ultimate goals or purposes; (2) the substance of public health: a statement about subject matter; (3) the organizational framework of public health: a statement that distinguishes the concerns included in the term "public health" from the ways in which society organizes to deal with them.

Figure 4-5 is a diagram of how the conceptual elements of the public health vision relate to one another. The governmental institutions have unique authority, obligations, and duties. Public health as a government responsibility considers: (1) 1. the duties that are essential to government's responsibility for public health; (2) the expression of these duties at the central or federal, state, and local levels; (3) the relationship between government and the private sector.

By separating the organizational expression of public health from understandings of its mission and subject matter, the committee intends to emphasize that the goals and concerns of public health can and should be addressed not only by health departments, but also by private organizations and practitioners, other public agencies, and the community at large. The governing role of the official public health agency in assuring that the overall system works is, however, indispensable.

4.2.2 Definition of Public Health System

The IOM emphasizes that public health extends beyond government and encompasses, "the efforts, science, art, and approaches are used by all sectors of society (public, private, and

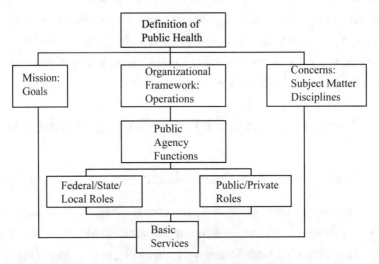

Figure 4-5　Conceptual Elements of Public Health Proposed by IOM

civil society) to assure, maintain, protect, promote, and improve the health of the people"①. The IOM defines six critical "actors" who are in a position to greatly affect health: communities, the health care delivery system, employers and business, the media, academia, and government.

Public health systems are commonly defined as "all public, private, and voluntary entities that contribute to the delivery of essential public health services within a jurisdiction". These systems are a network of entities with differing roles, relationships, and interactions. All of the entities within a public health system contribute to the health and well-being of the community or state.②

Other definitions of public health also emphasize the collaboration between the public and private sectors in the organization and activities of public health. Van Wave, Scutchfield, and Honoré (2010) assert that: the public health system is defined as the collective resources, infrastructure, and effort of all public, private, and voluntary entities and their respective roles, relationships, and interactions that contribute to the delivery of essential public health services to the population within a jurisdiction. The CDC states: "The governmental public health agency—both at the state and local levels—is a major contributor and leader in the public health system, but these governmental agencies inannot provide the full spectrum of Essential Services alone." (CDC, 2007). The IOM (1988) defines the public health system as the "activities undertaken within the formal structure of government and the associated efforts of private and voluntary organizations and individuals". Further, the IOM (2003) finds that a public health

---

①　Committee on Assuring the Health of the Public in the 21st Century, 2002:20.

②　Centers for Disease Control and Prevention [CDC], 2007.

system is a complex network of individuals and organizations that have the potential to play critical roles in creating the conditions of health. They can act for health individually, but when they work together toward a health goal, they act as a system—a public health system.

Although there is much to recommend this broader understanding of the public health system, it is also too extensive for an introduction. In this chapter, we will focus on the governmental public health system, with some attention to the private actors who frequently collaborate with it (e.g., academia, nonprofit health organizations, professional associations). The decision to focus on government is, in part, practical: taking an especially broad view of the public health "system", which encompasses a multitude of actors in all areas of society— largely without any formalized organization, relationships, or roles-renders it largely resistant to generalization, and as we will see, the governmental system is itself sufficiently complex all on its own. Governmental public health agencies constitute the backbone of the public health system and bear primary, legally mandated responsibility for assuring the delivery of essential public health services. Therefore, the role of government in assuring the nation's health is one that must be continued and sustained (IOM, 2003). Government is also key because "public health" functions, at least in large part, are to provide for people who are not suitably or effectively provided for by the private sector.

4.2.3 Organization of Public Health System: Examples from the United States

The governmental public health system in the United States is comprised of several departments and agencies within the federal government, at least one state-level agency for every state and territory in the country, and approximately 2800 local health agencies. Hundreds of thousands of public health workers staff these agencies, including Association of State and Territorial Health Officials (ASTHO, 2008), U.S. Department of Health and Human Services (DHHS, 2009); National Association of County and City Health Officials (NACCHO, 2009). Given our cognitive preference to find order in systems and our predispositions about the structure of organizations, it may be tempting to imagine from this rudimentary description that the U.S. public health system is a centralized, cohesive, hierarchically arranged organization in which the federal government sets policy and marshals resources, which it then distributes to the states, which in turn establish the infrastructure for implementation of those polices and provision of public health services to the population through local health departments, which then deliver them.

In truth, however, the governmental public health system in the United States is highly decentralized. The federal government has little direct control over state public health matters. States are generally responsible for their own public health systems, and in most circumstances, states delegate at least some of that authority to local political units—cities, towns, counties, and so forth—which set and implement their own public health policies. Rather than exercising authority over health matters in the United States, the federal government's role is primarily one influence. This influence is broadly either of the "persuasive" variety, whereby research and recommendations conducted at the federal level inform the decisions of more local public health policymakers and actors, or of the "financial" variety, whereby the federal government provides financial support to state and local public health agencies, frequently on the condition that the funds be used in a particular manner. The limited authority the federal government does have is generally restricted to those issues that have been recognized as affecting commercial or business conditions across state lines. Thus, the U.S. government public health system is a highly complex system of discrete, often independent, decentralized, and varied agencies. The decentralized and largely local character of the public health system is, in substantial part, a consequence of the legal, political, and historical context in which the public health system developed and operates. Largely, the organization of the public health system and the delivery of public health services can be traced to the principles of federalism governing the broader political and governmental organization of the United States (Turnock & Atchison, 2002). Under the U.S. federal system, sovereign power is shared between the federal government and the states, with certain powers delegated to the federal government exclusively, certain powers retained by the states exclusively, and some powers held by both the federal and state governments (subject to the limitations of federal supremacy).

4.2.3.1　Federal Government

Two developments since the founding period laid the groundwork for the enormous expansion of federal government health activity in modern times. Firstly, the Supreme Court decision in McCulloch v. Maryland set out the doctrine of implied powers, which expanded the potential powers of the national government beyond those specifically delegated in the Constitution to those reasonably implied by the delegated powers. (McCulloch v. Maryland, 1819) Secondly, the passage in 1913 of the Sixteenth Amendment authorizing a national income tax, substantially expanded the federal revenue- raising capability.

The commerce clause, interpreted under the doctrine of implied powers, and the power to tax for the general welfare under the Constitution have been the primary bases for much of national government health activity. Under the commerce clause, the Congress has the power to regulate commerce affecting more than one state, including health aspects of commerce. Federal grants-in-aid to states and localities in support of the general welfare have enabled the federal government to influence state- and local-health activity in line with national priorities. In addition, the federal government provides technical advice and assistance to states.

A long era of expansion in the federal role began in the 1930s and continued through the Great Society period of the 1960s. During the following decade the tide turned, and a nationwide redirection of emphasis emerged. This trend has decreased the federal presence in health, among other policy areas, and resulted in increasing reliance on state- and local level activity and funding. Despite the relative deemphasis on national government action, the federal role remains crucial. A primary activity is overall health policy development for the nation, including a variety of efforts to focus nationwide attention on major public health problems and encourage action on the part of other levels of government and of private groups. Such efforts may appropriately include provision of funds, but the potential for federal health policy leadership extends far beyond what can or should be expressed in dollars.

Federal leadership in public health issues is particularly critical if national scientific and professional expertise is to play its proper role in the policy process, offsetting the influence of special interests that tend to be especially decisive in smaller-scale public affairs. Public health's knowledge base is the core of what it has to offer to protect the health of the American people, and this knowledge depends on national government advocacy in order to function most effectively. The federal government also plays an irreplaceable role in the development of national health data and in the conduct of research.

4.2.3.2 State Government

Under the Constitution, the states are the repositories of powers not specifically delegated to the federal government. They have the primary responsibility for the well-being—including the health—of their citizens, and have exercised their powers over the years in a multitude of ways: they are the constitutional source of local government authority and can delegate broad powers over health matters to county and municipal governments.

The marked expansion of federal activism beginning in the Franklin D. Roosevelt presidency and the huge increase in intergovernmental fiscal transfer programs during the 1960s and 1970s added greatly to state responsibilities without removing existing ones. At the same time, because conventional policy wisdom was critical of state administrative capability and skeptical of some states' willingness to fulfill national priorities, many federal funding programs bypassed state governments entirely. Today, despite increased state activities and despite considerable efforts in the states to reform governance processes, according to the Advisory Commission on Intergovernmental Relations, "it does seem that improvements in state governmental performance have not been matched by a commensurate increase in their role as independent polities and policymakers" (Advisory Commission on Intergovernmental Relations, 1985).

The key ingredients of state role include:

(1) Statewide assessment, policy development, and assurance. It is the state's responsibility to see that functions and services necessary to address the mission of public health are in place throughout the state. This can be done by encouraging, providing assistance to,

and/or requiring local governments or private providers to perform certain of these functions. The state may also elect to provide certain services directly.

(2) Designating a lead agency for public health in the state (the place of ultimate responsibility) to fulfill the functions of assessment, policy development, and assurance. In most cases this will be the state health department, which has the obligation—and should have the authority—to ensure that important public health policy goals are being met, even when their implementation has been assigned to another entity.

State primacy in public health presents an opportunity for the entire nation to benefit by learning from evaluations of innovations and variations in public health programs at the state level.

4.2.3.3 Local Government

The vast numbers, overlapping jurisdictions, and varying authority of local governments make generalization difficult. Service responsibilities and fiscal capabilities are heterogeneous, and often the unit obligated to provide a service is not responsible for its financial support. From the public health perspective, perhaps the central problem is that our three-level model of government, placing basic responsibility for the people's health at the state level, does not fit well with the reality that health services must be delivered locally.

The strengths of local governments for the provision of public health are as follows: (1) serve as a governmental presence at the local level, ensuring each citizen's access to the security, protection, and authority of government; (2) provide a mechanism for implementation and integration of a complex array of needed services; (3) perform these functions on the basis of both professional and community-specific knowledge and in line with community values to the extent that they are consistent with the maintenance of individual rights; (4) convey information on local needs, priorities, and program effects to the state and national levels.

4.2.4 Financing Public Health

Funding for the public health system is mainly from public sources: taxes and other monies, such as fees, collected by the government at the different levels. For the developing countries, donation is also an option for public health financing. The total expenditure for the public health system in 2008 is estimated by the CMS as $69.4 billion in the united states , of which $10.4 billion came from the federal government and $59 billion from state and local government (CMS, 2010). These figures do not include some important public health services. Government spending for public works, environmental functions (air and water pollution abatement, sanitation and sewage treatment, water supplies, and so on), emergency planning and other such functions are not included.

4.3 Public Health System Performance Evaluation

4.3.1 Accountability and Evidence Based Public Health

Evaluation of the public health system is increasingly important in this era of accountability and finite budgets. Like the health care system, the public health system's performance is generally evaluated on three criteria: (1) effectiveness, (2) efficiency, and (3) equity (Aday, Begley, Lairson, & Balkrishnan, 2004; Aday, Begley, Lairson, & Slater, 1993). Therefore, the overall evaluation of public health performance asks the question: how effective, efficient, and equitable is public health in achieving its mission to prevent disease, injury, disability, and premature death by "assuring conditions in which people can be healthy"?

Effectiveness focuses on whether the desired benefits of public health practices—programs, policies, services—are achieved. Efficiency focuses on how the benefits achieved by public health compared to the resources expended to realize them, and whether alternate practices would have achieved greater benefits or the same benefits using fewer resources. "Equity addresses the fairness and effectiveness of policies in minimizing population health disparities" (Aday, 2005). The effectiveness, efficiency, and equity criteria are often complimentary. Improving effectiveness while holding resources constant increases efficiency, and those increases in efficiency may create opportunities for improved effectiveness and equity. These criteria—effectiveness, efficiency, and equity—provide a basis for evaluating the performance of the public health system, as they do for evaluating the health care system.

The movement to evaluate public health performance, systematically, has resulted in the need to substantiate what works and what does not work in public health practice—evidence-based public health—based on scientifically valid empirical research. We explicitly seek to base our initiatives, programs, and policies aimed at preventing disease, injury, disability, and premature death in populations on knowledge that has resulted from sound researches is about the effectiveness, efficiency, and equity of public health practices. As Kohatsu and his colleagues write, "Decisions and policies in public health are frequently driven by crises, political concerns, and public opinion. A number of researchers, however, are proposing a more evidence based approach to public health, based on the advances of evidence-based medicine" (Kohatsu, Robinson, & Torner, 2004).

The logic of evidence based practice identifies a cyclic relation between evaluation, evidence, practice, and further evaluation. It is based on the premise that evaluations determine whether anticipated intervention effects occur in practice, and identify unanticipated effects. The reports of such evaluations are valuable sources of evidence to maximize the benefits, and reduce the harms, of public health policy and practice. The evidence can also inform evaluation planning, and thus improve the quality and relevance new research.

Evidence-based public health is an activity with direct parallels to evidence-based medicine. The goals and general methods are the same, although some of the specifics differ because of the differences between medicine and public health. As some authors have noted, public health is a broader, more diverse field, and therefore a wider range of scientific approaches is needed to gather information for practice improvement. Kohatsu et al. (2004) have identified differences between evidence-based medicine and evidence-based public health.

In general, performance evaluation takes place at two levels: (1) the individual program, policy, or service level; or (2) the population level using population mortality and morbidity measures where these global measures are used to assess macro-level performance. Evidence-based public health usually refers to the program, policy, or service level.

4.3.1.1　Framework of the Evaluation at the Individual Program, Policy, or Service Level

Evaluations at the level of specific programs, services, or policies have identified goals that are targeted at defined populations. Therefore, measures of effectiveness, that is, measures that indicate whether the desired or intended result was brought about, are population and program specific. The basic components of any evaluation—program or system—are structure, process, and outcomes. When assessing a program, service, or policy, structure refers to the resources available to the public health program including organization and financing; the characteristics of the populations targeted by the program, service, or policy; and the physical, social, and economic environments in which the program occurs. Process refers to the implementation of the public health program, service, or policy. Outcomes refer to the expected results of implementation. Program-specific outcomes usually consist of short-term goals, such as a change in knowledge and attitudes; longer term goals, such as a change in behavior; and impact, such as a change in health status. Each of these goals would be specific to the program and the targeted population. The two most useful concepts are process and outcomes evaluations. "Process evaluations focus on the degree to which the program has been implemented as planned and on the quality of the program implementation. Process evaluations are known by a variety of terms, such as monitoring evaluations, depending on their focus and characteristics". Outcome evaluations, often used interchangeably with impact evaluations, focus on whether the goals of the program, service, or policy have been achieved and whether the changes desired can be attributed to the program. Table 4-1 shows a typical framework of evaluation for public health program.

Table 4-1   **Framework of Evaluation for Hypertension Intervention Program**

Structure	Process	Outcome
System Characteristics **Multi-organizations** **Access and convenience**	*Technical Style* Information pushing Recording & Tracking Email and E-diary Discuss group	*Clinical End Points* Blood pressure control
Provider Characteristics **Multidisciplinary team** **Specialty training**	*Interpersonal Style* Active specialist & GP interaction Active patient & physician interaction Peer support	*Health status* *Health behavior* *Self-Efficacy*
Patient Characteristics Demographic Social-economic Hypertension Co-morbidities	*Support service* Health education Symptom management Drug Management Psychological coping skills	*Health Resource* Health utilization Direct cost
Support Strategies **Tailoring** **Group Setting** **Feedback** **Psychological emphasis** **Medication counseling**		

4.3.1.2   Indicators for the Evaluation at Population Level

Population level indicators are often the measure of impact of a program, service, or policy. These include population mortality and morbidity rates. Historically, population health indicators have been age-adjusted death rates, disease-specific death rates, life expectancy, time lost to premature death, and infant mortality rate (IMR). The United Nations International Children's Emergency Fund's (UNICEF) definition of IMR is the probability of dying between birth and exactly 1 year of age (UNICEF, 2010). This rate is expressed per 1000 live births per year. IMR is an important measure that indicates the well-being of infants, children, and pregnant women, as it is associated with maternal health, quality and access to care, and public health in a given population. Life expectancy is defined by the World Health Organization (WHO) as the number of years of life that can be expected on average in a given population.

By using the life expectancy within that population, the time lost to premature death, also called years of potential life lost or YPLL, can be calculated. YPLL indicates that death occurred at an age less than what would be expected, and the more premature a death, the greater the loss of life (WHO, 2006a). A more recent concept of population health takes into account quality of life. Healthy life expectancy (HALE) at birth is defined by WHO as the "average number of years that a person can expect to live in 'full health' by taking into account years lived in less than full health due to disease and/or injury" (WHO, 2006a). HALE is a measure that "combines length and quality of life into a single estimate that indicates years that can be expected in a specified state of health" (Kindig, 1997). Other health-adjusted life expectancy measures are quality-adjusted life years (QALY), which emphasizes the individual's perceived health status as the indicator of quality of life; disability-adjusted life years (DALY), which combines mortality and disability measures; and years of healthy life (YHL), which combines perceived health and disability activity limitation measures from the National Health Interview Survey (Kindig, 1997).

Mortality rate is the number of deaths in a given population per year (WHO, 2006a). The age-adjusted mortality rate takes into account the population's age distribution when calculating mortality rate. Using a statistical method that "standardizes" the target population to a reference population, this measure is commonly used when comparing mortality rates across different populations.

4.3.2   Methodological Design for Public Health Evaluation

The three major types of study designs for public health evaluation are: randomized experiments, quasi-experiments, and non-experimental designs. Several factors differentiate one design from another:

(1) Whether a "control" or "comparison" group is used. A control or comparison group is a group of persons, facilities or communities similar to those who receive an intervention but who have not been exposed to the intervention. The purpose of a control or comparison group is to provide an estimate of what would have happened if you had not implemented.

(2) How participants are assigned to intervention and control group. In some evaluation studies, participants are assigned to intervention and control groups through random assignment. In others, control groups are selected rather than randomly assigned to match the characteristics of the intervention group, with the exception of their exposure to the intervention being evaluated.

(3) The timing of data collection in relation to program implementation. An evaluation may collect data before, during and/or after program implementation

(4) The complexity of statistical analysis required. Some study designs require a more highly sophisticated statistical analysis.

4.3.2.1   Randomized Experiments

Randomized experiments have the highest degree of validity among the evaluation designs. In evaluations using this study design, participants are assigned by chance (i.e., randomly) to a group that will receive an intervention (called the intervention group) or to a group that will not receive the intervention (called the control group). The two main types of randomized experiments are pretest-posttest control group designs and posttest-only control group designs.

Pretest-posttest control group design follows these steps: (1) randomly assign persons, facilities or communities to experimental groups; (2) take measurements both before and after the intervention; and (3) measure impact as the difference between changes in outcome indicators for the intervention group and the control group.

Posttest-only control group design follows these steps: (1) randomly assign persons, facilities or communities to experimental groups (same as pretest-posttest control group design); (2) take measurements only after the intervention; and (3) measure impact as the difference between outcome indicators for the intervention group and the control group, at some point after program implementation.

4.3.2.2 Quasi-experiments

Quasi-experiments use similar experimental groups, selected through non-random methods. If it is not feasible to randomly assign experimental groups, you can still take into account many of the external factors affecting your control and intervention groups by using a quasi-experimental design. This can be done by choosing a control group that is as similar as possible to the intervention group, often by matching on characteristics that are considered to be important antecedents of the outcomes sought by a program. The three most commonly used types of quasi-experiments are: non-equivalent control group pretestposttest design, non-equivalent control group posttestonly design, and generic control design.

Non-equivalent control group pretest-posttest design follows these steps: (1) create experimental groups by matching particular characteristics that are considered to be important antecedents of the outcomes sought by the program; (2) take measurements both before and after the intervention; and (3) measure impact as the difference between changes in outcome indicators for the intervention group and the control group.

Non-equivalent control group posttest only design follows these steps: (1) create experimental groups by matching particular characteristics that are considered to be important antecedents of the outcomes sought by the program; (2) take measurements only after the intervention; and (3) measure impact as the difference between outcome indicators for the intervention and control groups, at some point after program implementation.

Generic control designs can be used to assess whether changes or trends in outcome indicators for young adults exposed to your program differ from those in the general population of young adults. For example, imagine that you want to compare program data and national survey data regarding condom use among young adults. Using a generic control design, you might find that the proportion of your program target audience who used condoms in their last sexual encounter had increased significantly over the course of your program but was still lower than the national level recorded among young adults.

4.3.2.3 Non-experimental Designs

Non-experimental designs do not use control or comparison groups. For this reason, these designs are a generally weaker means of measuring program impact than experimental designs. Nonexperimental designs are used when: (1) you have not made provisions for a control or comparison group as part of the evaluation plan, (2) a program or intervention is expected to reach the entire target population; (3) this type of program is often referred to as a full-coverage program. These designs include time-series design, pretest-posttest design and posttest-only design

4.4 Meta-leadership in Public Health

To achieve public health objectives, public health will need to serve as leader and catalyst of private efforts as well as performing those health functions that only government can perform. Weak and unstable leadership cannot deal with the inherent complexity in public health practices. To tackle this complexity, we need leaders whose scope of thinking, influence, and accomplishment extends far beyond their formal or expected bounds of authority. Such leaders can be called as meta-leaders. "meta-leadership" refers to guidance, direction, and momentum across organizational lines that develops into a shared course of action and a commonality of purpose among people and agencies that are doing what appears to be very different work.

These broad analytic themes of meta-leadership can be translated into the five dimensions: (1) the person of the leader and his/her awareness or problem assessment; (2) the problem, change, or crisis which compels response; (3) leading one's entity and/or operating in one's designated purview of authority; (4) leading up to bosses or those to whom one is accountable; and (5) leading cross-system connectivity. The meta-leader operates along these five domains of action, variably leveraging each dimension of thinking and practice as called for by circumstances, and always having these different yet complementary perspectives at hand. See figure 4-6.

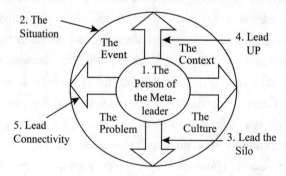

Figure 4-6   Five Dimensions of Meta-leadership in Public Health Practices

4.4.1 The Person

Personality, experience, culture, emotional expression, and character are significant factors in the conduct and impact of meta-leaders: the "who" of the construct (Kirkpatrick &

Locke, 1991; Trompenaars, 1994). And yet, these very individual and personal qualities vary significantly from leader to leader. Knowing that many different personality types can achieve the mantle of meta-leader, what common qualities distinguish those able to from those unable to achieve such far-reaching influence? Meta-leaders tend to be "big thinkers." These are people willing to take a large and complex problem and—with courage and fortitude in hand—search a wide expanse for solutions. They have abundant curiosity and prolific imagination to contemplate and activate that which has not been otherwise discovered (Sternberg, 2006, 2007). They are integrative strategists, charting a course that allows stakeholders to operationally link and leverage one another in order to accomplish shared objectives. And most importantly, sometimes against the odds, they have a penchant and capacity for making meaningful things happen.

Meta-leaders also possess what is referred to by Daniel Goleman as "emotional intelligence" (Burns, 1979; Goleman, 1996). People who direct large scale or complex initiatives must convey these attributes: (1) self-awareness; (2) self-regulation; (3) motivation; (4) empathy; and (5) social skills. Because they are watched and challenged by audiences beyond their usual social circles, meta-leaders must be comfortable in their own surroundings, in the milieu of others, and must have the talent to make other people feel comfortable and assured. The self-discipline, drive, understanding, and capacity to form meaningful and satisfying relationships are critical in the effort to cross the usual divides and boundaries of organizational, professional, and cultural association.

4.4.2 The Situation

Finding the most appropriate solution to a problem or response to a crisis depends first on precisely determining what is occurring (Bransford & Stein, 1993; Pretz, Naples, & Sternberg, 2003). This is a difficult task because there is often—if not always—a gap between objective reality and subjective assessment (e.g., Hazleton, Cupach, & Canary, 1987). This is more likely to occur when many different people and organizational units are involved, when a great deal of information is required to diagnose the problem, when the stakes and emotions are high, and when the analysis and action are time constrained. In other words, the greater the complexity, the more difficult it is to develop a factual, evidence-based, clear, and actionable description of what is occurring. This objective though elusive depiction of reality is at the heart of dimension two of meta-leadership.

To understand the complexities of dimension two is to grasp the disparities between what one believes to be true and the actual truth (Mullin, 2002). This is a particularly cogent problem in the midst of an unfolding crisis. In a volatile and quickly changing scenario, the gap is inevitable, since it takes time for information to emerge and assessments to evolve. In practice, this requires the meta-leader to grasp, to work with, and to narrow that likely reality-belief gap, aided by the collection of further information, the passage of time, and the perspective of hindsight. Such complex circumstances demand the capacities and skills for strategic "situational awareness" (e.g., O'Brien & O'Hare, 2007). the connectivity between the personal capacities and understandings embedded in meta-leadership dimension one and the realities of the situation that are addressed in dimension two.

The meta-leader has the perspective and measured patience to work with ambiguity. If the situation was clear and every action had a certain and predictable cause and effect, the skills and aptitude of the meta-leader likely would not be called into action. However, crisis situations, high consequence organizational predicaments, and difficult inter-personal conflict each by their nature do not come with clearly obvious computations for what is right and what is wrong (Slaikeu, 1998). Not everyone faced with these ordeals is equally able to establish a calculated assessment and then rise to the challenge: these are among the strategic and analytic capacities uniquely associated with the meta-leader.

4.4.3   Lead the Silo

In complex environments—typified by multiple organizations, departments, and units operating in overlapping domains-those people who arise as meta-leaders rarely operate as independent actors: they have their own organizational base of operations within which followers see them in charge (Phillips & Loy, 2003). In that entity, the leader carries authority, has resources at his or her disposal, and functions within a set of rules and roles that define expectations and requirements. Those subordinates expect adherence to allegiances and loyalties, trusting that the leader will advocate on behalf of their best interests (Heifetz, 1999). In bureaucratic terms, these accomplishments are often measured in expanding resources, authority, or autonomy for the entity and its members. In many bureaucratic settings, departments and divisions compete amongst one another, and followers expect their leaders to triumph on their behalf (Lee & Dale, 1998).

The meta-leader is a leader of leaders, and fosters leadership development throughout the system, though first at home among his or her constituents. Leadership, after all, does not reside with one person. In robust organizations, it is embedded among many people and at multiple levels of the hierarchy (Northouse, 2004). Meta-leaders drive the leadership learning curve-effective leadership is a continuous learning process-encouraging those who work under their supervision: building, marshalling, and communicating a vision and a message that is as a group developed, executed, assessed, and persistently adjusted and improved as contingencies require. The meta-leader fosters meta-followership within his or her entity: proactive thinkers and doers who are able to greatly expand and inspire the impact which they together seek to achieve. Doing this requires a sense of leadership confidence and security: strong, smart, capable followers are not seen as a threat but rather as a vital asset (Sternberg, 2007). In this way, the meta-leader seeks "dogs that hunt": empowered people who share the passion, commitment, instinct, and capacity to get things done.

4.4.4 Lead Up

Most people who work in organizations have a boss. The chief executive officer(CEO) of a publicly traded corporation has the board of directors. Below the CEO are a series of subordinates who serve as boss to their staffs. Government agencies have strict supervisory oversight. And even the President, Governor, or Mayor must account to their electorates. Embedded in the culture of this country—founded as a rebellion to the monarchy—is a reluctance to invest too much power or authority in any one person to avoid its being exercised for abusive or inappropriate purposes. As a result, our culture has in both its public and private sectors a complex system of checks, balances, and oversights to limit autonomy and autocracy.

How is this leading up accomplished? The great meta-leader is a great subordinate: dependable, honest, reliable, and loyal. He or she validates the power and command equation, respecting and serving the objectives and proclivities of those in charge. In so doing, the meta-leader crafts vertical connectivity and bi-directional feedback. Influence is shaped by informing and educating his or her boss. Bosses of course vary in style and temperament, and the meta-leader appreciates that as with any relationship, this is one that must be carefully and strategically managed (Marcus et al., 2006). When this works well, the boss appreciates the prioritization and management of problems and decisions: the focus is on the truly important questions that are worthy of his or her time, thereby reducing distractions. In shaping that focus, the meta-leader intentionally and transparently communicates information and a variety of reasonable options in order to craft strategic assessment and solution building. The great subordinate manages assumptions, does not promise what cannot be delivered, and assures that the boss is never surprised. This last point is a sensitive matter. While bad news and valid criticism are hard to deliver, the meta-leader practices "truth to power": anticipating and managing the dangers and distractions of explosive problems. In the best circumstances, complements balance criticisms, and both are equally welcomed when honest and deserved (Kotter, 1999).

There is another important aspect to the fine art of leading up. What if the boss engages in immoral, illicit, or dangerous activity with the expectation that followers will do just that: accept without questioning? Herein reveals a moral responsibility for followers (Smiley, 1992). Just as the check and balance system works from boss to subordinate, so too must it at times function from subordinate to boss (Kellerman, 2004). Being a good subordinate does not imply passive compliance with inappropriate, unlawful, destructive behavior: it is not blind loyalty. It also at times requires the subordinate to draw the line, bypass immediate leaders and lead up above them, or at the extreme, to demonstrate the courage to resign.

4.4.5 Lead Across

In building a wide sphere of influence, the meta-leader grasps that just as vertical, "up-down" linkages are important, so too are horizontal linkages. By leveraging the capacity of many adjacent centers of expertise and capacity, the meta-leader is able to engage the spectrum of agencies and private interests that are to be recruited to a shared enterprise (Ashkenas et al. , 2002). This is the value-added of the meta-leader: the ability to generate a common, multi-dimensional thread of interests and involvement among entities that look at a problem from very different yet complementary vantage points. By combining their assets and efforts, the meta-leader envisions and activates more than what any one entity could see or do on its own.

Why is this both important and difficult? Often, wide social problems and questions demand the engagement of a wide set of constituencies. These different groups and entities will not, on their own, recognize the lines of influence and capacity which they could generate together. In fact, they might very well see themselves in competition with one another: if credit or benefit falls to one entity more than another, the noble purposes can be undermined by those who question "what's in it for me?" The meta-leader is able to focus attention on the shared purposes while at the same time tempering those forces of suspicion and jealousy that constrain their achievement (Marcus et al. , 2006).

How is this accomplished? The meta-leader is keen to identify and understand the individual intrinsic motives of these different stakeholders and constituencies in generating a connectivity of thinking and action. The job is in aligning these disparate yet complementary cognitive spheres into a unified plan of action. Each entity must be recognized for its unique profile of interests, experiences, and contributions to the shared enterprise. While it is common for people to focus upon the differences and conflicts among them, the meta-leader turns the attention to points of agreement: shared values, aspirations, objectives, and circumstances. With a new appreciation for their points of commonality, stakeholders are able to creatively envisage what they could accomplish if they were to join forces, building new equations and strategies of common ground and achievement. The meta-leader knows actions speak louder than words, and early triumph is a critical factor in demonstrating the value added of working together.

Cohesion of action cannot begin in the moment of decision and action: it must be embedded into the thinking and activity of agencies and people, a purpose and mission upheld by the meta-leader (Daft, 2005). It is akin to crafting gears whose inter-linking teeth and shapes are carefully formed: when it is time to move, the cogs link in a way that ensures movement and not stasis. For this reason, designing cross-system connectivity of action is a strategic and methodological building endeavor, by which both the process and outcome of the effort attest to the value and benefits of working toward common purposes. As stakeholders experience the advantages of leveraging the knowledge, resources, and expertise of others, and as they recognize the benefit and added influence gained when their contributions are likewise leveraged by others, the efforts and connectivity generated by the meta-leader builds a momentum of its own: impact and collaborative value both arise and thrive. Even so, the meta-leader recognizes that to keep the connected effort on track, it must be carefully monitored and adjusted; so it perseveres beyond the expected bumps and challenges; and so that it remains current with new developments and demands.

The meta-leadership model described here emerged out of observation and analysis of difficult times. The United States and the world were reeling from the unprecedented events of 9/11, the devastating failures of the Hurricane Katrina response, and the specter of further crises that could rock the foundations of society. It also emerged out of the triumphs and failures of leadership at the time: the difficulties in getting organizations and people to work together when that connectivity of action was the best hope for mounting an effective response; the inspiration and results when communities, businesses, and public agencies joined forces to accomplish what otherwise would have been inconceivable.

The meta-leadership model speaks to the complex web of values and beliefs that have shaped this country and others around the world. This is a culture that cherishes the competitive spirit along with the independence and freedoms afforded individuals and entities to pursue what they—in the wide realm of what is legal and appropriate—see fit to do. It also values limits on power that ensure that no government official or company executive will be able to abuse their authority for illicit or corrupt purposes. And finally, it appreciates what can be accomplished when people come together, rally, and overcome daunting obstacles.

In that complex web, extraordinary leaders emerge, able to balance those values and beliefs by virtue of their strength of character and keen analytic skills along with their ability to lead, follow, and engage others. They forge both impact and collaboration that would not have otherwise been achieved. These meta-leaders—who certainly predate this model that seeks to describe them—deserve further study so that their important work and contributions can be better appreciated and understood, better supported, and taught to others.

Chapter 5   Community Health Care

5.1   Introduction

This chapter introduces the concepts and characteristics of community health, explains the importance of community health care, describes how to conduct community health assessment, and provides a brief review of community health care in China.

5.1.1   Community Health

5.1.1.1   Health

Different people used the word "health" to mean very different things, and there is no universally accepted definition. However, the most widely quoted definition of health was the one adopted by the World Health Organization (WHO) in 1946 at the International Health Conference, and this definition was entered into use in 1948. WHO defines health as "a state of complete physical, mental and social well-being and not merely the absence of disease or infirmity". The Definition has not been amended since its inception①. Since health is ever-changing, it is also defined as a dynamic state and encompasses a continuum from well-being to disease.

Many factors combine together to affect the health of individuals and communities. The context of people's lives determine their health, and individuals should not be blamed for poor health. These determinants include income and social status, education level, physical environment where we live, social support networks, genetics, health services, gender, and etc. These above factors do not act in isolation. Rather, they interact and interconnect. All these factors have considerable impacts on health, whereas the more commonly considered factors such as access to and utilization of health care services often have less of an impact②.

---

① Preamble to the *Constitution of the World Health Organization* as adopted by the International Health Conference, New York, 19-22 June, 1946; signed on 22 July 1946 by the representatives of 61 States (Official Records of the World Health Organization, no. 2, p. 100) and entered into force on 7 April 1948. http://who.int/about/definition/en/print.html

② http://www.who.int/hia/evidence/doh/en/.

5.1.1.2 Community

There is no consensus regarding the definition of community. A community is often thought of as a geographic area with clear boundary. Some scholars regard community as a group of people who have common characteristics. Therefore, communities can be defined by location, race, ethnicity, age, occupation, interest in particular problems, outcomes or common bonds. A community may be as large as all of the individuals who make up a nation (even all the people in the world) or as small as the group of people who study in a class in a school.

It is important to clearly defining community relative to health and health care, because it will identify the target population for action of healthcare service providers and identify the availability and access to services for community members.

5.1.1.3 Community Health and Public Health

We defined community health as the health status of individuals and groups in defined community and the actions and conditions to promote, protect, and preserve their health. Community health, public health, primary health and some other terms (e.g. population health, global health) were usually used interchangeably by laypeople and professionals who work in the health domains. Public health is the most inclusive, and it is the science and practice of preventing disease, promoting population health, and extending life through organized local and global effort.

Primary health and Community health are overlapped term. As for primary health, WHO & UNICEF defined its eight essential components at the Alma-Ata Conference in 1978①, and they are: (1) education for the identification and prevention/control of prevailing health challenges, (2) proper food supplies and nutrition; adequate supply of safe water and basic sanitation, (3) maternal and child care, including family planning, (4) immunization against the major infectious diseases (5) prevention and control of locally endemic diseases, (6) appropriate treatment of common diseases using appropriate technology, (7) promotion of mental, emotional and spiritual health, (8) provision of essential drugs. Primary health care is essential health care based on practical, scientifically sound and socially acceptable methods and technology made universally accessible to individuals and families in the community through their full participation and at a cost that the community and country can afford to maintain at every stage of their development in the spirit of self-reliance and self-determination. It forms an integral part both of the country's health system, of which it is the central function and main focus, and of the overall social and economic development of the community. It is the first level of contact of individuals, the family and community with the first element of a continuing health care process(WHO,1978, Article VI). Primary health care was regarded as the key to attaining

---

① WHO & UNICEF. The Alma-Ata Declaration, 1978.

the goal Health for All by the Year 2000.

　　Community health is influenced by various determinants acting and interacting of four levels: personal and family level (e. g. genetic endowment, health behaviors, and socioeconomic status), community level (e.g. societal environment, culture and acculturation, physical environment, and health care), societal level (e.g. policies and politics, population movements, and demographic transition), and global level (e. g. climate change, globalization, and communications)①. Practitioners, policy-makers, and researchers should take a broad view of the determinants of community health. The relationships among the different levels may vary in different communities and different populations, which implied the relationships should be identified before improving a defined community health and its health care.

5.1.2　Meaning of Community Health Care (CHC)

　　Although currently, more attention and expense are paid to the healthcare delivery and medicines in nearly all the countries, people gradually find the economic, social determinants and individual behaviours are more critical to health than the healthcare system and utilization of healthcare. There are some reasons why community health care (or community-based health care, community-oriented health care, CHC) was paid more attention to than before.

　　Firstly, the disease and death spectrum has been changed from the middle of 20th century globally. The infectious diseases (e.g. tuberculosis, measles, and malaria) are no longer the main cause of death; on the contrary, more deaths were caused by noninfectious diseases (e.g., cancer, diabetes, heart diseases, and malignancies). According to the report of WHO, noncommunicable diseases were responsible for 68% of all deaths around the world in 2012, up from 60% in 2000. The 4 main noncommunicable diseases are cardiovascular diseases, cancers, diabetes and chronic lung diseases②.

　　Secondly, global aging entails community health care. According to the United Nations' definition, an ageing society is one in which more than 7% of the population is over the age of 65 or more than 10% of the population is over the age of 60. Population aging is one global trend in the 21st century. For example, The share of people 65 and older in the total population in the countries of Europe and Central Asia (ECA) rose from 6 percent in 1950 to 12 percent in 2015③. The seniors were susceptible to a variety of chronic diseases, and would need more community health care because of limited self-care ability.

---

　　① Gofin Jaime, and Gofin Rosa. Essentials of Global Community Health. Jones and Bartlett Learning, 2011.

　　② http://www.who.int/mediacentre/factsheets/fs310/en/index2.html.

　　③ Bussolo Maurizio, Koettl Johannes, and Sinnott Emily. Golden aging: prospects for healthy, active, and prosperous aging in Europe and Central Asia. World Bank Publications, 2015.

Thirdly, community health care is more efficient health resources allocation & control medicine costs. Figure 5-1 shows that there are three levels of healthcare. They are:

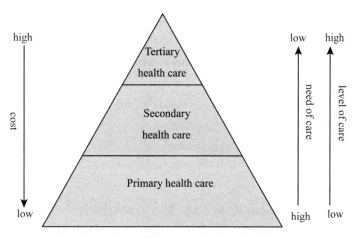

Figure 5-1 Three Levels of Health Care

(1) primary health care: it is the "first" level of contact between the individual and the health system where essential health care is provided. A majority of prevailing health problems can be satisfactorily managed. It is generally provided by the primary health institutions or General Practitioner/ Family Doctor.

(2) secondary health care: curative services were provided and more complex problems are dealt with, and it is provided by the district hospitals.

(3) tertiary health care: it offers super-specialist care and is provided by regional/central level institutions.

In comparison with hospital-based healthcare, community health care is more cost-effectiveness especially in a broad view. And it is a strategy to attain primary health.

5.1.3 Characteristics of CHC

Now, let's elaborate on the characteristics of CHC.

5.1.3.1 Primary Care

CHC often provides quality, basic and essential health services, and these healthcare covers from health promotion to the end of life care. As mentioned above, it is generally provided by the primary health institutions or General Practitioner/Family Doctor (they work as gate-keepers).

5.1.3.2 Preventive Care

Health promotion/education is conducted to educate, influence, and motivate them to make good health decisions. Meanwhile, CHC often covers immunization and disease prevention program. For example, in China, community health service centers in the urban areas and township hospitals in the rural areas are generally in charge of the immunization program.

5.1.3.3   Comprehensive, Continuous, and Coordinate Care

Comprehensiveness of care means that care is provided for all types of health problems. Continuity of care requires that the management of a patient's care over time be coordinated among providers. And coordinate care generates genuine service integration and coordination between deferent health care, e.g. referral service.

5.1.3.4   Accessible Care

CHC is reachable and convenient services. To the community residents, CHC is not only with good geographic and economic accessibility but also with cultural accessibility.

5.1.3.5   Personalized Care

CHC Focuses on the person not the disease.

5.1.3.6   Family as a Vital Unit of Care, Community-oriented Care

Besides the individuals, CHC is concerned with the family structure & function, and regards a family as a vital unit of care.

CHC is community-oriented care, which means it addresses most important problems in a defined community since different communities have their own features and health priorities.

5.2   Community Health Assessment (CHA)

Before we conduct community health care or relative activities, we should know clearly about the health status of community. Community Health Assessment (CHA) is a dynamic and ongoing process undertaken to identify the strengths and needs of the community, establish the health priorities, and facilitate collaborative action planning directed at improving community health status and quality of life.

CHA includes three processes. Firstly, it is a technical process. CHA often uses analytical tools and technologies to generate and evaluate evidence. Secondly, CHA is a social process because it needs to invite participation from citizens and health care providers in decision making. Thirdly, CHA should deal with issues of the worth of health and life, societal fairness, and resource priorities, which will be involved an ethical process.

5.2.1 Some Models for CHA

There are some models for CHA that have been created by governmental agencies and professional association for special projects or programs.

5.2.1.1 Healthy Cities/Health Communities (WHO)

Healthy Cities/Health Communities is an initiative of WHO, and this model or project has been implemented widely around the world.

"A healthy city is one that is continually creating and improving those physical and social environments and expanding those community resources which enable people to mutually support each other in performing all the functions of life and in developing to their maximum potential." (WHO, 1998) ①

Healthy Cities/Health Communities is a framework rather than a prescription. There is no step-by-step instruction for employing it. How to implement it depends on the community, and the issues the community wants to address, and the values and capacities of the groups and individuals in the community. There are, however, some basic components of any Healthy Cities/Health Communities initiative:

(1) Generate a compelling vision, and this vision should be based on values shared among all participants and on a high quality of life for everyone in the community values, and it may be broad or more specific.

(2) Embrace a comprehensive view of health and well-being both at the individual level and at the community level and acknowledge the social determinants of health (such as peace, shelter, education, food, income, a stable ecosystem, sustainable resources, social justice, and equity that The Ottawa Charter lays out) and the interrelationship of health with these issues.

(3) Engage citizen participation and seek community ownership. All citizens themselves from different racial, ethnic, and socio-economic groups and all walks of life should originate, plan, and implement any community initiative. And all sectors of the community (such as government, health care, education, the business, target populations, ordinary citizens and etc.) should be represented in an initiative, and the community should feel that it creates the initiative, owns it, and control its direction.

(4) Address quality of life for all and address issues through collaborative problem-solving. A Healthy Cities/Health Communities initiative should be aimed at improving the quality of life for all individuals and groups. People should be encouraged and helped to work together to reach creative solutions to disagreements and conflicts.

(5) Focus on systems change not on individual problems.

---

① WHO. Health Promotion Glossary. 1998. WHO/HPR/HEP/98. 1. http://www. who. int/entity/healthpromotion/about/HPR%20Glossary%201998.pdf? ua=1.

（6）Build capacity using local assets and resources. All these individuals, groups, businesses, institutions, governments and resources should be joined in pursuit of a common vision.

（7）Track progress and outcomes.

5.2.1.2　Mobilizing for Action Through Planning and Partnerships（MAPP）

Mobilizing for Action through Planning and Partnerships（MAPP）is a strategic planning tool for community health improvement developed by the National Association of County and City Health Officials in U.S.A.

MAPP consists of multiple steps in six phases（Figures 5-2）. In the first phase, Organize for Success/Partnership Development, core planners decide whether the MAPP is timely, appropriate, and even possible. If it does, an inclusive committee composed of keys stakeholders is created.

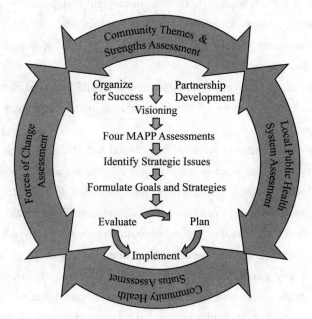

Figure 5-2　Mobilizing for Action Through Planning and Partnerships

In the second phase, the community develops a shared vision of health in the community and common values that guide the planning and action to follow.

Source: Reprinted with permission from the National Association of County and City Health Officials, MAPP Framework, Copyright ©2016. Used with permission.

In phase 3, the Four MAPP Assessment, is the main feature and strength of MAPP model. These are four interconnected assessments are: （1）the community themes and strengths assessment (assessing of community opinion and identifying of community assets), (2) the local public health system assessment (LPHSA) (general capacity of the local health department), (3) the community health status assessment (the health of community members and of the community as well as the quality of life issues such as employment, housing, the environment, etc.), and (4) the forces of change assessment (forces such as legislation, technology, and other issues that do or will impact on community health).

In phase 4, Identify Strategic Issues, a prioritized list of the key issues is identified based on assessment data. Only issues that must be addressed in order to realize the shared vision are considered.

In phase 5, Formulate Goals/Strategies, sets goals and formulates strategies for reaching those goals.

Finally, in phase 6, the Action Cycle, comprises the planning, implementation, and evaluation of the action. This process is ongoing and it continues until the community achieves its vision … and generates a new vision to work toward.

There some other models of CHA, such as PRECEDE/PROCEED (PRECEDE stands for Predisposing, Reinforcing, and Enabling Constructs in Educational/Environmental Diagnosis and Evaluation and PROCEED stands for Policy, Regulatory, and Organizational Constructs in Educational and Environmental Development), Community as a Partner, and etc.

5.2.2 Recommendations Concerning CHA

Although these above-mentioned models or approaches have their own characteristics, it should be noted that they have same features. Here are some recommendations where we carry out for CHA:

(1) CHA is guided shared vision and values. Keep the vision and values at the forefront throughout the CHA process.

(2) CHA is a process. It involves the community in reviewing the data, identifying problems, setting priorities, developing an action plan, monitoring progress, assess whether the actions are effective, modifying the plan if necessary, and reevaluating the community's problems and priorities. One problem is solved, and a renewed CHA is needed to identify the next problem. CHA isn't a one-time endeavor but ongoing cycle.

(3) Participation of all community members. In the process of CHA from identifying problems to assess effectiveness and to move on to the next problem, all citizens from different groups, all walks of life, and all sectors of the community should participate. Especially for the stakeholders and partners, when particular issues are identified and the solution involves specific individuals or groups.

(4) Develop an action plan, implement it, and measure progress. The goal of CHA is to address the problem in the community. If CHA does not bring any action, then it is not worth doing. Once the plan is implemented, use data to determine whether the actions are having the

desired effect, if not, find out why and change the plan.

(5) Make use of information. Utilize data to help the community to identify problems, set priorities, track progress, and change the plan if necessary.

5.3　Health Care System and CHC Delivery in Mainland China

CHC can be traced back to 1930s. In 1997, the term "community health" firstly appears in national governmental document *Decision of the Central Committee of the Communist Party of China and the State Council Concerning Public Health Reform and Development*(《中共中央、国务院关于卫生改革与发展的决定》(中发〔1997〕3 号).) It should be noted that some primary and community health services were provided by the basic health institutions before.

The former Ministry of Health and nine other Ministries distributed *Some Suggestions on Urban Community Health Service Development*(《关于发展城市社区卫生服务的若干意见》(卫基妇发〔1999〕326 号)) in 1999, The former Ministry of health and ten other Ministries distributed *Suggestions on Speeding Up the Development of Urban Community Health Services* (《关于加快发展城市社区卫生服务的意见》(卫基妇发〔2002〕186 号)), and the *State Council distributed the Guiding Suggestions on Urban Community Health Service Development* (《关于发展城市社区卫生服务的指导意见》(国发〔2006〕10 号)) in Feb of 2006. From then on, China's community health services have developed greatly.

As the CHC network, there were 8669 community health services (CHS) centers and 25569 CHS stations by 2014. Table 5-1 displays the status of CHS in China.

Table 5-1　　　　　　　　　**Community Health Services in China**

Year	2014	2013
Street (number)	**7696**	**7564**
CHS center (number)	**8669**	**8488**
bed (number)	171754	167998
Health Personnel (number)	381856	368636
#Health Professionals(number)	323053	311332
#Registered Doctor & Assistant Doctor(number)	134258	130907
Visits (100 Million)	5.4	5.1
Inpatients(10 000)	298.1	292.1
Daily Visits Per Doctor (number)	16.1	15.7
Daily Inpatients Per Doctor (number)	0.7	0.7
Utilization of Beds (%)	55.6	57.0
Average Length of stay (day)	9.9	9.8

续表

Year	2014	2013
CHS stations（number）	**25569**	**25477**
Health Personnel（number）	106915	107437
#Health Professionals（number）	94450	94886
#Registered Doctor & Assistant Doctor（number）	42740	42931
Visits（100 Million）	1.5	1.5
Daily Visits Per Doctor（number）	14.4	14.3

Source: the National Health and Family Planning Commission.

CHS institutions（including centers and stations）provide prevention, health care, basic medical service, rehabilitation, health education, and family planning advice. For example, the functions of prevention involved the prevention and control of infectious diseases, endemic disease and parasitic diseases（including immunization schedule）, prevention and cure of chronic diseases, health supervision, etc.

Chapter 6　Burden of Disease(BOD)

6.1　Background and Professional Terms of BOD

6.1.1　Background of BOD?

6.1.1.1　Play a Text of Burden of Disease

Write down all cost you paid for your health service (outpatient, inpatient, preventive health, excluding supplement) in last year? $x_1 = ?$

- How many days you were in beds or missing class? $x_2 = ?$
- How many days your friends or classmates company you in order to look after you? $x_3 = ?$
- How much you are willing to pay for one day or daily wage? $x_4 = ?$
- How much your friends are willing to pay for one day or daily wage? $x_5 = ?$
- $y = x_1 + x_2 \cdot x_4 + x_3 \cdot x_5$

6.1.1.2　True Story: SARS in China 2002—2003

SARS (severe acute respiratory syndrome) is a deadly pneumonia-like disease that appeared in China in 2002 and spread across China and into Southeast Asia and North America in the winter and spring of 2003, killing several hundred people, scaring many more and disrupting economies and travel plans around the world. (see Table 6-1 and Table 6-2)

Table 6-1 **Direct Economic Burden of SARS in Guangzhou**

Economic burden(CNY)	sample	Average exp.(CNY)	proportion(%)	Total expense *
In-patient exp.	1059	20263.21	83.66	25997698.43
Outpatient exp.	339	463.43	1.92	594580.69
Recovery exp.	339	848.27	3.59	1088343.24
Drug exp.	339	2646.91	10.59	3395985.53
total		24221.83	100.00	31076607.89

* Taking 1283 clinic cases as example to estimate total expense.

Table 6-2   **Indirect Economic Burden of SARS in Guangzhou 2003**

Burden of disease	Male	Female	Total
Premature death	6874607.32	8019734.14	14894341.46
Losses in production	2603091.94	3171702.18	5774794.12
Total	9477699.26	11191436.32	20669135.58

Between November 2002 and July 2003, SARS in southern China caused an eventual 8273 cases and 775 deaths reported in many countries with the majority of cases in Hong Kong (9. 6% fatality rate). According to WHO. Within weeks, SARS spread from Hong Kong to infective individuals in 37 countries in early 2003 (cases from 1 November 2002 to 31 July 2003, WHO).Questions for you:

(1) How did SARS influence society?

(2) How did SARS influence social economy?

(3) How did SARS influence human beings?

(4) And how can we compare it with Ebola outbreak in Africa in 2014?

The WHO is aiming to ensure that the number of new cases of Ebola disease, and it does not rise to more than 10000 cases a week by the beginning of December 2014 and then starts to fall.

The goal is part of a new program introduced by the United Nations Mission for Emergency Response, which aims that within 60 days from mid-October 70% of new infections will be isolated and 70% of burials will be safe. And within 90 days the goal is that the number of new infections will be decreasing in 80% of areas affected by Ebola disease.

WHO's director general, Bruce Aylward, told a telephone press conference that at 14 October there had been 8914 cases of Ebola disease, including 4447 deaths, but that the numbers would continue to rise over the next few months (see Table 6-3).

Table 6-3   **Filoviridae Virus Occurrences in the World**

Viral species	Year of discovery	Geographic origin	Number of outbreaks	Number of human cases	Number of deaths(CFR)	CPR(%)
Marburg Marburgvius	1967	Uganda	4	465	145	31
Sudan ebolavius	1976	Sudan	6	792	426	54
Zalve ebolavius	1976	DR Congo	12	1388	1100	79
Reston ebolavius	1989	Philippines	0	0	0	—
Tal forest ebolavius	1994	Cote Devoir	0	1	0	—
Bund bugyo ebolavius	2007	Uganda	2	208	78	38

CFR: case fatality rate.

Disease burden is the impact of a health problem on a given area, and can be measured using a variety of indicators such as mortality, morbidity or financial cost. This allows the burden of disease to be compared among different areas for example regions, towns or electoral wards (see small area analysis section). It also makes it possible to predict future health care needs.

6.1.2   Terms of Burden of Disease(BOD)

(1) burden of disease(BOD) means the total loss of future years of disability free life that are lost as the result of the premature deaths or causes of disability occurring in a particular year. In other words, the burden of disease is a measurement of the gap between the current health of a population and an ideal scenario where everyone completes their full life expectancy in full health.

(2) Economic burden of disease means the total economic lost as result of the case, disability and premature for individual and society. How can we convert it?

(3) Economic burden of disease can be measured from different perspectives: Society, population or individual.

In 1993, economic burden of disease in China got to 320.8 billion CNY, represented 9.3% of GDP for 1993; in 2003, this figure reached 120 billion CNY, accounted for 10.3% of GDP for 2003 . The growth rate of economic burden of disease was faster than the rate of GDP development(about 9%).

Chinese people are confronted with double burdens of disease including communicable disease(ADIS,SARS,TB and hepatitis B) and non- communicable disease(malignant tumors, injury and intoxication, diseases of circulatory)

Non-communicable diseases were the leading cause of burden of disease in China now(see Table 6-4).

Table 6-4   **Rank of Burden of Disease**

	Individual	Household	Society
1	stroke	AIDS	AIDS
2	tumors	Mental disorder	Hepatitis B
3	injury	injury	Mental disorder
4	TB	tumors	TB
5	Mental disorder	stroke	tumors
6	diabetes Mellitus	TB	stroke
7	Hepatitis B	Hepatitis B	injury
8	AIDS	diabetes Mellitus	diabetes Mellitus

Note: How can we measure and compare burden of disease fairly and rationally?

6.1.3 Index to Measure Burden of Disease

6.1.3.1 Case Index

(1) Incidence: A measure of morbidity based on the number of new episodes of illness arising in a population over a period of time.

It can be expressed in terms of sick persons or episodes per 1000 individuals at risk. For example: Incidence of HBP = 10/1000 in 2013 of Wuhan City, how can we get it?

(2) Prevalence: A measure of morbidity based on current sickness in a population, estimated either at a particular time (point p.) or over a stated period.

It can be expressed either in terms of affected people (persons) or episodes of sickness per 1000 individuals at risk. Two-week prevalence rate is a common index to measure the prevalence, see Table 6-5 as an example.

Table 6-5   **Two-week Prevalence Rate in China**

Year	Total (%)	Urban (%)	Rural (%)
2008	18.9	22.2	17.7
2003	14.3	15.3	14.0
1998	15.0	18.7	13.7
1993	14.0	14.5	12.8

Source: The Fourth National Health Services Survey in China, 2008.

6.1.3.2 Death Index

(1) Mortality Rate: The number of deaths in the population divided by the average population (or the population at midyear)

(2) Standardized Mortality Rate (Adjusted Mortality Rate): The age-standardized mortality rate is a weighted average of the age-specific mortality rates per 100000 persons, where the weights are the proportions of persons in the corresponding age groups of the WHO standard population.

(3) Maternal Mortality Rate (MMR): The number of maternal deaths related to childbearing (from pregnancy to 42 days after delivery) divided by the number of live births in that year.

(4) Maternal Mortality Rate (see Figure 6-1):

① Deliveries at home and deliveries without skilled attendants.

② Complex array of socio-economic, environmental, and cultural factors that contribute to high maternal mortality:

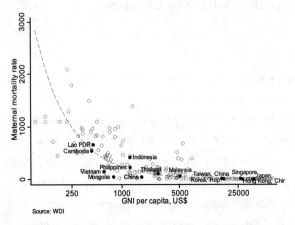

Source: WDI

Figure 6-1   Maternal mortality rate vs income, 2005

Low social status of women;

Malnutrition;

Unequal access to health care resources.

(5) Infant Mortality Rate(IMR): The ratio of the number of deaths among children less than one year old during a given year to the number of live births during the same year. It is probability of dying between birth and age 1 per 1000 live births, which reflects the level of mortality, health status, and health care of a population, and the effectiveness of preventive care and the attention paid to maternal and children health.

(6) Premature Death: The difference between actual age at death and life expectancy at that age in a low-mortality population.

(7) Life Expectancy: The number of years a person would be expected to live, starting from birth (for life expectancy at birth) and similarly for other age groups, on the basis of the mortality statistics for a given observation period.

Infant Mortality Rate is widely used indicator of the health of a population. Life expectancy measures quantity rather than quality of life.

What do you think is the current under 5 mortality rate in the following countries (number of deaths < 5 years / 1000 live births)?

(8) Potential Years of Life Lost (PYLL): The number of years of life "lost" when a person dies "prematurely" from any cause - before age of life expectancy (life expectancy in China is 70).

Potential years of life lost are calculated by taking the median age in each age group, subtracting from 70, and multiplying by the number of deaths in that age group disaggregated by sex and cause of death(see Table 6-6).

$$PYLL = \sum_{i=1}^{n} a_i d_i \qquad a_i = 70 - j_i$$

a_i—70 minus the median age in i^{th} age group;

d_i—Numbers of death in i^{th} age group;

j_i—the median age in i^{th} age group.

Table 6-6 **PYLL Caused by Cerebrovascular Diseases in a Certain Area**

Age group	Median age	Number of death	Years of life lost	PYLL
0~	0.5	1	69.5	69.5
1~	3.0	0	67.0	0
5~	10.0	3	60.0	180
15~	17.5	2	52.5	105
20~	25.0	8	45.0	360
30~	37.5	49	32.5	1592.5
45~	52.5	265	17.5	4637.5
60~	67.5	707	2.5	1767.5
75~		969	0	0
Total		2004	—	8712

Deaths index gives us advantage:

① Allow comparing health interventions targeting the same problem;

② Allow comparing different diseases;

③ Does not take into account:

- Age at death;
- Disability.

6.1.3.3 Disability

In the context of health experience, a disability is any restriction or lacking (resulting from impairment) of ability to perform an activity in the manner or within the range considered normal for a human being (WHO 1980).

1. Disability Index

Four scenarios after illness:

(1) Recovery totally from acute sickness;

(2) permanent disability after suffering from illness, such as limping after polio;

(3) Death after a period of disability;

(4) Death soon after illness.

2. How to measure permanent or short-term disability;

(1) Endow weights according to severity of disability;

(2) Disability weights usually come from WHO or through consulting in different countries.

Age weights:

• One year lost does not have the same meaning according to the age

• Age weights attribute lower weights for:

Childhood;

Older age.

3. Discounting

(1) Yeas of lost do not have the same value if lost:

• Today (e.g., measles)

• Later (e.g., hepatitis B)

(2) Discounting rate:

• Rate that discounts the value each year;

• Apply to costs and effects, e.g. 3%;

• Subject to discussion:

Should DALYs be discounted?

At what rate?

Do we need other estimates of burden of disease?

• Both mortality rates and life expectancy are useful, but do not tell us anything about disease burden in people living with diseases

• They cannot be best captured by trying to assess quality of life

• Another option to express disease burden is in terms of loss of productivity

4. Disability-Adjusted Life Years (DALYs)

(1) Allow comparing health interventions targeting the same problem;

(2) Allow comparing different diseases;

(3) Take into account age at death;

(4) Take into account disability.

Measuring death and disability with the same metric (see Figure 6-2).

Disability-adjusted life years (DALYs):

(1) Comprehensive measure;

(2) Take into account loss due to:

• Death (Years of life lost, YLLs)

• Disability (Years lived with disability, YLDs)

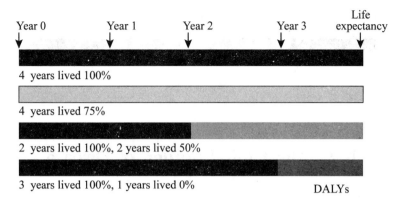

Figure 6-2

(3) The equivalence is:

- Death = 100% disability
- Perfect health = 0% disability

The equivalence between disability and death(see Figure 6-3).

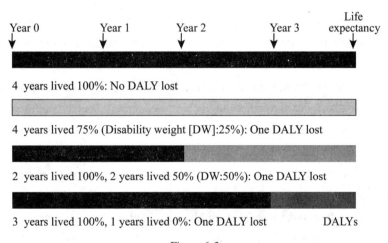

Figure 6-3

Calculating DALYs(see Figure 6-4):

(1) Calculate years of life lost through death;

(2) Calculate years of life lived with disability;

(3) Add the two.

1year lived 100%, 2 years lived 50%, 1 year lost, so there were 2 DALYs lost.

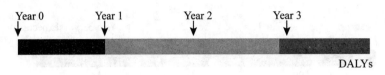

Figure 6-4

6.2   The Global Burden of Disease

6.2.1   Global Burden of Disease

There are some 6 billion people in the world, and hundreds of millions experience disease or injury each year. Taken as a whole, the combined pain, suffering, loss of productivity and unrealised hopes and dreams are our world's burden of disease.

In other words, the burden of disease is a measurement of the gap between the current health of a population and an ideal scenario where everyone completes their full life expectancy in full health.

The Global Burden of Disease project attempts to measure this total disease burden. The GBD study is collaboration between the WHO, the World Bank and the Harvard School of Public Health.

GBD is a measure of the amount of disease, disability, and death in the world today. It is a product of complex and interwoven demographic, economic, social, political, religious and environmental factors. It refers to the collective impact of disease on the world population.

Disease burden can be attributed to either *specific diseases* (e.g. HIV, TB, obesity, diabetes) or risks for health (unsafe sex, overcrowding, smoking, excess cholesterol). Therefore, the measurement of GBD allows us to address preventable diseases in each region of the world — how much of risks to health could be avoided in the future years.

An important development of this project was a single indicator of total disease burden — the DALY.

6.2.2   Disability-Adjusted Life Years (DALYs)

$$DALY = YLL + YLD$$

YLL means Years of Lost Life (due to premature mortality)

YLD means Years Lost to Disability (due to injury or illness)

The DALY is the internationally-accepted measure of death and disability and is increasingly cited as a powerful tool for decision makers in international health.

Calculation of DALYs is based on the assumption that everyone has a right to the best life expectancy in the world. The only differences in the rating of a death or disability should be due to age and sex but not income、culture、location or social class.

Sample "DALY" calculations for a disease

Example A: 100000 children are stricken for 1 week with a disease with a disability weighting[1] of 0.3; 2% die at 2 years old. (LE = 82 years), how many DALYs did they lose?

$$DALYs = YLD + YLL$$
$$= 100000 \times 7/365 \times 0.3 + 100000 \times 2\% \times (82-2) \times 1$$
$$= (100000 \times 7/365 \times 0.3) + (2000 \times 80 \times 1)$$
$$= 575 + 160000$$
$$= 160575$$

Example B: 100000 adults are stricken for 2 years with a disease with disability weighting[2] of 0.6; 20% die at age 80 years. (LE = 82 years), how many DALYs did they lose?

$$DALYs = YLD + YLL$$
$$= 100000 \times 2 \times 0.6 + 100000 \times 20\% \times (82-80) \times 1$$
$$= (100000 \times 2 \times 0.6) + (20000 \times 2 \times 1)$$
$$= 120000 + 40000$$
$$= 160000$$

6.2.3 Why Are DALYs Important?

DALYs attempt to provide an appropriate, balanced attention to the effects of non-fatal as well as fatal diseases on overall health. In the absence of such assessments, conditions which cause decrements in function but not mortality tend to be neglected.

DALYs help to inform debates on priorities for health service delivery, research and planning. For example, DALYs can be used to:

(1) Compare the health of one population with another—and allow decision makers to focus on health systems with the worst performance;

(2) Compare the health of the same population at different points in time;

(3) Compare the health of subgroups within a population—to identify health inequalities (see Figure 6-5 and Figure 6-6).

---

[1] There are STANDARDISED DISABILITY RATINGS for various conditions.
e.g. Deafness = 0.33, Down syndrome = 0.5, Diarrhoea = 0.12

[2] There are STANDARDISED DISABILITY RATINGS for various conditions.
e.g. Deafness = 0.33, Down syndrome = 0.5, Diarrhoea = 0.12

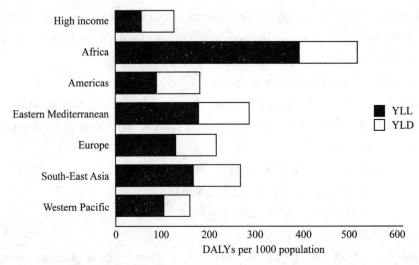

Figure 6-5   YLL, YLD and DALYs Lost by Region, 2004
Resource: Health Statistics and Informatics Department, WHO, 2009

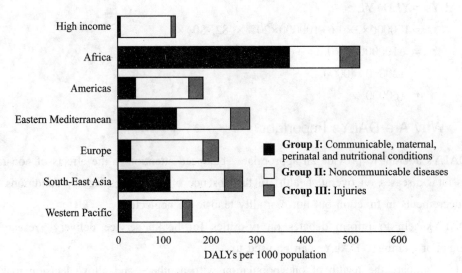

Figure 6-6   Burden of Disease by Broad Cause Group and Region, 2004
Resource: Health Statistics and Informatics Department, WHO, 2009

Table 6-7   **Comparison between Various Measures of Burden**

	Cases	Deaths	YLLs	DALYs
Allow comparisons for the same disease	✓	✓	✓	✓
Allow comparisons between diseases	✕	✓	✓	✓
Take age at death into account	✕	✕	✓	✓
Take disability into account	✕	✕	✕	✓

DALYs: Social values.

6.2.4 Disability Weights(DW)

(1) In GBD, non-fatal consequences of diseases and injuries understood as transitions through different "health states"

YLD calculation requires aggregate assessments of the overall decrements in health associated with particular health states → disability weights

DWs are measures of overall levels of health rather than contribution of health to overall welfare

(2) GBD 1990: DW elicited from panel of health professionals following explicit protocol evaluating 22 indicator conditions in an intensive group exercise with "deliberative phase" using person trade-off (PTO) method. Responses averaged across participants

(3) New Disability Weight Project:

The new DW will have a greater emphasis on paired comparisons, anchored by time trade-off methods.

It also aims to engage members of the general community (including those in developing countries) to a greater degree.

The DW project is being carried out in two stages:

(1) Community surveys: It's a community household survey in selected regions,

- Pemba, Bangladesh, Indonesia, Peru, USA;
- Cultural diversity >> representativeness;
- Paired comparisons.

(2) Internet survey: It's an online open-access survey.

- the primary source of data for the final DW;
- will include randomly selections from all 230 squeal;
- open to all interested in participating (open-access).

Includes a variety of measurements paired comparisons, ranking, visual analogue scale, time trade-off, population equivalence) to anchor the scale (paired comparisons, ranking, visual analogue scale, time trade-off, population.

6.2.5 Discounting

Discounting commonly practices in economic analyses. We assume that individuals value their health more now than at some point in the future. So in the future health loss occurs the more they are discounted(see Table 6-8).

GBD1990 used 3% discounting by most researchers in the world. There are some important issues:

age	Discounted YLL	Undiscounted YLL
0	30.3	80
25	27	55.5
40	23.5	40.6

Table 6-8　**Discounting by Age**

（1）Why discount?

（2）Consistency with cost-effectiveness analyses

（3）Prevent giving "excessive" weight to deaths at younger ages

6.2.6　Age Weighting

It is used to reflect a social preference that values a year lived by young adult more highly than that of young children or the elderly. An Australian survey found that respondents considered saving four 20-year olds as important as saving ten 60-year olds（see Figure 6-7）:

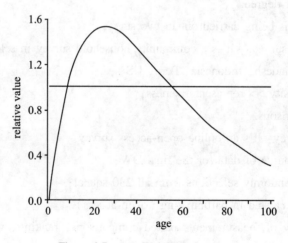

Figure 6-7　Age Weighting by Age

Not related to productivity but 'social' role in caring for the young and old people;

Age weighting,

Arguments against:

Unacceptable on equity grounds;

Does not reflect actual social values;

But, everyone potentially lives through every age→not inequitable.

6.3　Classification and Calculation of Burden of Disease

6.3.1　Direct Economic Burden and Indirect Burden of Disease

6.3.1.1　Direct Economic Burden

Direct economic burden is the total health expenditure for the disease prevention and treatment. Including:

(1) The expenditure for health service buying.

Outpatient, inpatient, recovery, medicine, etc..

(2) The expenditure for obtaining the health service and other relative activities.

Transportation, food and nutrition...

6.3.1.2　Indirect Economic Burden of Disease

Indirect economic burden of disease is the cost of labor time loss—The patient & relatives. Including: The cost due to labor time lost by pationts and their relatives, the expeaditure for transport, food, et al by patients' caregivers.

6.3.2　The Measurement of Direct Burden of Disease

6.3.2.1　Data Collection.

1. Direct medical expenditure collections

(1) Collect from the institutions—data is reliable and convenient to survey. However, cannot get the expenditure of a particular disease which you want.

(2) Collect from the patients—retrospective review survey or tracking survey.

(3) Self-buying medicine expenditure is belonged to this collection.

2. direct non-medical expenditure collections

The transportation, nutrition and food, etc.

6.3.2.2　The Estimate Method of Direct Burden of Disease

1. Top-down method

To obtain the total expenditure information of medical service of nation or region, then, divide it into patient groups in certain standard. However, we can't get any information about non-medical expenditure.

2. step-model method

Two step model: year medical expenditure = average in-patient expenditure of each time of two-week visit rate×26+... Outpatient expenditure ...×26. For example:

(1) Direct Expenditure of disease(X_i) = average direct expenditure of disease of the year×

region population×incidence(or prevalence rate).

(2) Total direct expenditure = $\sum X_i$.

6.3.3   Measurement of Indirect Economic Burden

6.3.3.1   Data Collection

Indirect economic burden is the financial loss of society which is caused by disease, death and disability, especially caused by effective work time and work capacity decreased.

6.3.3.2   Data Collection Methods

1. Retrospective review and tracking survey

2. Other data you may need to collect

We give formulation as follows:

$$\text{PYLL} = \sum_{i=1}^{n} a_i d_i \qquad a_i = 70 - j_i$$

- Average wage;
- GDP: Gross Domestic Production;
- GNP: Gross National Production;
- National income.

Method for Measuring: The key point is how to measure the effective working value of the day or a year.

(1) Present value approach: wage standards×loss of effective working time.

(2) Human capital approach:

- delay days×average national income/365;
- Time loss×average GDP OR PYLL×average GDP;
- Average GDP×DALYs×Productivity weight.

Different age-group population has different productivity weight, usually we use these values as follows Table 6-9.

Table 6-9   **Productivity Weight by Age Group**

Age group	Productivity weight (Barum)
0~14	0
15~44	0.75
45~59	0.80
>60	0.10

6.3.4 Contingent Valuation Method

How much money you'd like to pay for avoiding a certain disease?

6.3.5 Break-in Cost Method

Productivity loss = the recovery time of production

Something we should pay attention to time value and burden of disease reported by researches.

6.3.5.1 Time value

(1) Time is money, money has discount rate.

(2) Discount rate = interest rate, sometimes, usually using 3%.

(3) Present Value of BOD = $\sum_{i=0}^{n} \dfrac{B_t}{(1+i)^t}$.

B_t— the burden of years of t;

i — discount rate;

t — time(year);

$1/(1+i)^t$— discount rate.

6.3.5.2 Rationality of Disease Economic Burden

Sometimes, the rising of economic burden is not always because of "bad things happened". Some caused higher medical cost have been reported, such as:

(1) The new medicine has been invented, replaced the old one.

(2) The new technology.

(3) Inflation or the rise of price of commodity in society.

(4) The medical price adjustment.

(5) The rising of incidence & prevalent rate, new disease, such as HIV, SARS, etc.

6.3.5.3 The Issue on—Who Is Seeing the Doctor

We should correct some common bias or wrong methods, such as:

(1) In some area, population of people who goes to see a doctor is lower than the population of morbidity or illness.

(2) Representativeness of data: Some data can't answer all the questions, such as the data collected in one hospital.

(3) Comparability of data: If the burden measured by different methods, they can't be compared with directly.

Chapter 7   Health Financing and Universal Health Coverage

7.1   Basic Concept of Health Care Financing

In a narrow sense, health financing refers to the process that the government departments raise sufficient funds to support the development of health services in a certain social environment. It involves the financing channels, proportion and quantity, moreover, the allocation and use of funds are included in the wide sense.

7.1.1   Purposes and Functions of Health Financing

Figure 7-1 depicts several reasons for building health financing mechanism. Because the disease is uncertain, consumers can not predit the occurrence of disease, and the high cost of treatment may lead some households trapped in poverty.

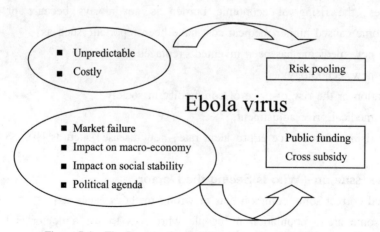

Figure 7-1   The Reasons for Building Financing Mechanism

There are three main purposes of health financing. Firstly, collect contributions efficiently and according to capacity to pay. Secondly, health financing aims to ensure access to service and financial protection for all individuals. Thirdly, we can set correct incentives for providers and make the best use of resources by health financing scheme. So, the above-mentioned purposes of the health financing settle on its function: revenue collection, pooling funds and purchasing services. There's one point which needs attention that government should find a balance between equity and efficiency and sustainability goals for health financing. The term sustainability indicates the extent to which a socially acceptable level of insurance coverage is affordable for everybody.

Generally, health financing is analyzed along three dimensions: revenue collection, pooling funds and purchase services. The chief aspect of health financing is revenue collection, which mainly refers to government tax authorities levy income tax on individuals and corporations according the capacity to pay (people with no financial capacity do not pay) and hand the operations of the pooled money over to social security agencies and health insurance agencies. Another function of health financing is taking advantage of the pooled funding to share risks, however, government tax authorities may pool funds at different levels and the scales and numbers will be different under different patterns, and risk resistance capacity varies with the scales of pools. The tax-based funding should be channeled to three directions: providers (Latin American countries)—to lower price services, insurance funds—to lower insurance premium, consumers (cash transfer)—to purchase services or insurance. The function of purchasing services will be introduced from two points of view: consumers side and provide side. A package of services which are necessary will be defined at the form view, and the content of services reflect national priorities. The audiences of health service and cost sharing also need to be unequivocal. When it comes to provider, we are usually concerned more about the nature of service provider, public or private. It is equally important that right incentives should be set to encourage health service provider to supply appropriate services with high quality and avoiding over provision, under provision and service with low quality.

7.1.2 Health Financing Schemes

Health financing scheme involves financing mechanisms and financing sources. Financing mechanisms mainly includes the following aspects: tax-based financing, social health insurance, out-of-pocket payments, and other prepayment schemes. (See Figure 7-2)

7.1.2.1 Tax-based Financing

The main form of tax-based financing is that the central and local department levy income tax on individuals and corporations. The indirect sources of revenue includes VAT、excise duties and import export tax, government-owned property and natural resource are also a large part of revenue in some developing countries. Tax-based funds mainly cover the cost of purchasing benefit package and social health insurance. Benefit package is normally not explicit, but often includes health prevention, MCH, essential treatment & drugs. Health department provides these services through public facilities for all population, especially for poor and other vulnerable. Public facilities are mainly funded through a budget. Incentives are set for provides, for example medical staff are paid by salary or a mix of payment methods.

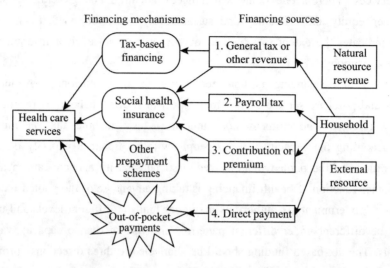

Figure 7-2   Payments of Health Care Services

7.1.2.2   Social Health Insurance

The revenue collection of social health insurance is derived from three aspects: compulsory membership with the household as registration unit, formal sector employees: payroll tax—proportional to income (ceilings often applied) shared by employee and employer, informal sector: flat rate or fixed rates for different population groups with government subsidies to disadvantaged population groups. Benefit package of social health insurance is clearly defined and cost sharing is applied. Fee-for-service or other payment methods are the common forms of payment of social health insurance.

7.1.2.3   Private Health Insurance

The revenue collection of private health insurance mainly comes from the voluntary membership, premium are flat rate, community-rating, individual-rating. But risk selection and adverse selection may exist in the private health insurance. Benefit package purchased is clearly defined, cost sharing is applied. Services are from public or private providers, private health insurance agencies may provide services directly. Private health insurance usually plays substitute, complementary and supplementary roles for public schemes.

7.2   Universal Health Coverage

7.2.1   The Meanings of Universal Health Coverage

The goal of universal health coverage is to ensure that all people obtain the health services they need without suffering financial hardship when paying for them. For a community or country to achieve universal health coverage, several factors must be in place, including: A strong, efficient, well-run health system that meets priority health needs through people-centred integrated care; A system for financing health services so people do not suffer financial hardship when using them. This can be achieved in a variety of ways; Access to essential medicines and technologies to diagnose and treat medical problems; A sufficient capacity of well-trained, motivated health workers to provide the services to meet patients' needs based on the best available evidence. It also requires recognition of the critical role played by all sectors in assuring human health, including transport, education and urban planning.

7.2.2 Impact of Universal Health Coverage

Universal health coverage has a direct impact on a population's health. Access to health services enables people to be more productive and active contributors to their families and communities. It also ensures that children can go to school and learn. At the same time, financial risk protection prevents people from being pushed into poverty when they have to pay for health services out of their own pockets. Universal health coverage is thus a critical component of sustainable development and poverty reduction, and a key element of any effort to reduce social inequities. Universal coverage is the hallmark of a government's commitment to improve the wellbeing of all its citizens. Universal coverage is firmly based on the WHO constitution of 1948 declaring health a fundamental human right and on the Health for All agenda set by the Alma-Ata declaration in 1978. Equity is paramount. This means that countries need to track progress not just across the national population but within different groups (e.g. by income level, sex, age, place of residence, migrant status and ethnic origin).

7.2.3 The Vision of Universal Coverage

Under universal coverage, there would be no out-of-pocket payments that exceed a given threshold, of affordability—usually set at zero for the poorest and most disadvantaged people. The total volume of the large box in is the cost of all services for everyone at a particular point in time. The volume of the smaller yellow box shows the health services and costs that are covered from pre-paid, pooled funds. (See Figure 7-3)

The goal of universal coverage is for everyone to obtain the services they need at a cost that is affordable to themselves and to the nation as a whole.

7.2.4 Universal Coverage and Health System

Some factors such as inequalities in income and education, social exclusion associated with factors: gender and migrant status remove some groups of people outside the health system. There are five important factors that will affect the function of health system (Figure 7-4), and financing mechanism is one of those factors. Weak health systems includes insufficient health

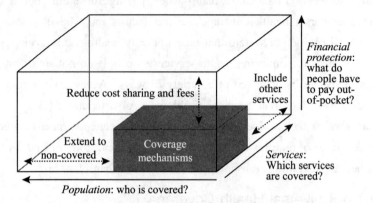

Figure 7-3 Measuning progress towards universal health coverage in three dimensions
(Source: World Health Organization and Busse, Schreyogg & Gericke)

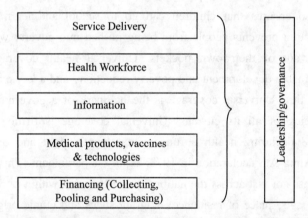

Figure 7-4 System Building Blocks or Functions

workers, medicines and health technologies, ineffective service delivery, poor information systems and weak government leadership may also hamper the process of universal health coverage. And the other parts cannot function if the financing system is weak.

7.2.4.1 Where We Are?

Some figures and diagrams may help us understand how far we are away from the universal health coverage. More than 1 billion people cannot use the health services they need. Around 150 million suffer financial catastrophe each year and 100 million are pushed into poverty because they need services, use them, but must pay at the time of use. Based on a conservative estimate, 20% ~ 40% of resources spent on health are wasted.

7.2.4.2 Inefficiency

Figure 7-5 depicts ten main factors leading to inefficiency of health system, such as spending too much on medicines and health technologies, using them inappropriately, using ineffective medicines and technologies; Leakages and waste, again often for medicines; Hospital inefficiency particularly over-capacity; De-motivated health workers, sometimes workers with the wrong skills in the wrong places; An inappropriate mix between prevention, promotion, treatment and rehabilitation.

1. Medicine: underuse of generics and higher than necessary price.
2. Medicine: use of substandard and counterfeit medicines.
3. Medicine: inappropriate and ineffective use.
4. Products and services: overuse/supply of equipment, diagnostic services and procedures.
5. Health workers: inappropriate or costly staff mix, unmotivated workers.
6. Health services: inappropriate hospital admission and length of stay.
7. Health services: inappropriate hospital size and low use of infrastructure.
8. Health services: medical errors and suboptimal quality.
9. Health system leakages: waste, corruption and fraud
10. Health intervention: inefficient mix and inappropriate level.

Figure 7-5　Ten Leading Sources of Inefficiency, WHR 2010
(Source: World Health Report 2010)

7.2.5　Regional Health Financing Strategy

Figure 7-6 offers some methods that will enable the governments to raise sufficient funds. The most frequently used method is increasing the efficiency of revenue collection. Efficiency is particularly important under a definite total amount of health funds. Besides the methods above, innovating financing mechanism and developing assistance for heath may both improve the level of capital. Figure 7-6 indicates the proportion of health expenditure in GDP in some South-East Asian countries.

7.2.6　Government Spending on Health in Defferent Countries

Figure 7-7 shows us the proportion of heath expenditure in total government expenditure of different countries. The proportion of health expenditure varies significantly among different nations. Solomon Islands has one of the world's highest percentages which exceeds 25%. While, the proportion in some countries may be below 10%.

7.2.7　Prepayment and Pooling

To collect more health financing and increase the degree of universal health coverage,

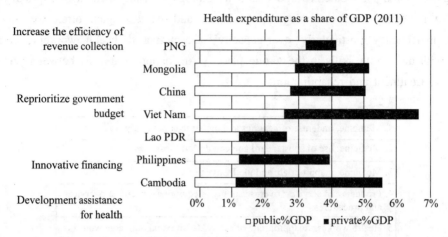

Figure 7-6　Raise Sufficient Funds

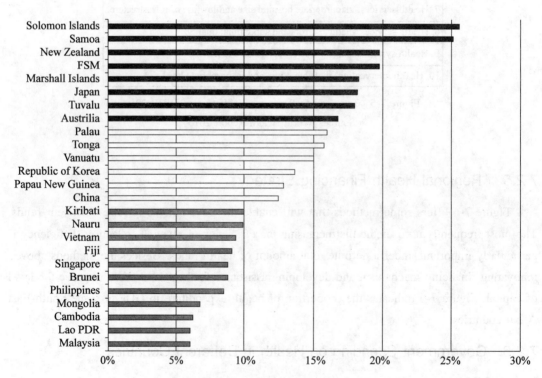

Figure 7-7　Government Priority to Health

(Source：World Health Report 2010)

countries choose different mechanisms, mostly a mix of tax-based funding with forms of insurance. Community insurance and micro-insurance can play a valuable role—particularly in the early stages. The compulsory contribution is another important aspect, it is difficult to ensure universal coverage without making contributions (taxes and/or insurance) compulsory. If the rich and the healthy opt out, the poor and sick are left with sub-standard services from the limited funds that remain. At the same time, a problem that we can not neglect is that where pools are fragmented, equity goals are much more difficult to achieve—the well paid and the elite obtain better benefits and are reluctant to share with others.

7.2.8 Protect the Poor and Vulnerable, and Improve Equity

Special attention needs to be paid to the poor and vulnerable in all systems, even when most funds are prepaid and pooled. So at certain context we should provide free or subsidized services (e.g. through exemptions or vouchers) for specific groups of people (i.e. the poor) or for specific health conditions cash payments to cover transport costs and other costs of obtaining care to reduce some financial barriers for the poor. Sometimes these are paid only after the recipient taking actions, usually preventive, that are thought to be beneficial for their health or the health of their families.

7.3　Social Health Insurance

7.3.1　Social Health insurance—History and Coverage Expectations

Social health insurance first established in Germany at the end of the 19th century and spread in Europe, it extended rapidly both in Europe and other regions after 1945. Now the universal coverage of social health insurance has achieved in many OECD countries. Expectations that with economic development, formal employment and social health insurance membership grows, but high rates of jobs in developing countries are in the informal economy. Social health insurance schemes generally cover only a small part of the population in developing countries.

7.3.2　Social Health Insurance and Coverage

Social health insurance has strongest potential for covering civil servants and workers in employment relationships of a certain level of formality. As a result, it will lead to difficulties in covering informal economy workers due to designed characteristics of social insurance. There are some population groups most often excluded outside social health insurance: self-employed workers, workers in small companies, agricultural workers, domestic workers, workers in the "informal economy", family helpers, non-employed family members and dependents.

7.3.3　Reasons for Exclusion—basis for Developing Extension Strategies

Characteristics of certain population groups(contributory capacity, priorities and interests) may be the main reason for exclusion. Factors such as administrative capacities, legal environment, insufficient public information may prevent some groups of people from being covered by social health insurance. And these reasons are the basis for developing extension strategies.

7.3.4   Strategies to Extend Coverage Through Social Health Insurance Schemes

Some certain strategies are came out to extend the coverage. One of them is to bring the health care into existing security schemes. Because many social security schemes offer old-age, disability, survivor pensions and work injury benefits but no health protection. But it may be a complex process due to the complexities of health care. Health care are very different from pension benefit administratively and financially. Contracting and other elements in the provision of health care are key factors that will condition the effort to reach.

The second strategy (classical method) is increasing extension of existing social health insurance schemes by providing coverage to new population groups and dependents of scheme members. The pace of this process is linked to development of administrative capacities. Transition to universal coverage will take long time. In Germany, it takes 127 years, Belgium is 118 years, Austria is 79 years, Japan is 36 years, Korea is 26 years. Rapid extension of coverage usually occurs at the beginning. Then, it takes long time to reach higher percentage. Government commitment, economic growth, solidarity within society, structure of the economy, labor force distribution and development of health system are influential factors that should be paid attentions in the incremental strategies.

Another effective strategy is that combating non-compliance and contribution evasion. Non-compliance will undermine solidarity and legitimacy even cause financial problems and informalization of employment. Reasons for non-compliance must be studied clearly in order to increase compliance and contribution collection. The attitudes of government towards evasion and political considerations might be the key reasons for non-compliance. From the view of individuals, myopia, low contributory capacity and low legitimacy also lead to non-compliance. Non-compliance are also aggravated by the factors at the employers side, including cost savings, low reputation costs and interests contradictions between employers and the government regulations. On the other hand, there are many factors that could help increase compliance and contribution collection such as government commitment, resources for enforcement and existing penalties, strengthen administrative capacities and degree of automation. Reducing transaction costs for collection by automation and simplification of administrative procedures for difficult-to-cover groups is also an effective measure.

The forth strategy is allowing existing social health insurance institutions to innovate. Much progress can be made through initiatives by existing social health insurance institutions. Some of the specific measures we have taken include improving administrative capacities and working towards good governance, working with existing organized civil groups. Administrative capacities can be improved by the following ways: improving efficiency, client focus and responsiveness, optimizing performance measurement, adoption of modern ICT tools.

7.3.5 Coherent and Integrated Social Protection Strategies

Finally, the above-mentioned strategies should be coherent and integrated with social protection strategies. Stakeholder support, coherency of individual policies are necessary to adapt in accordance with trend towards integrated and coherent social protection extension strategies. Horizontal strategies ought to be combined with vertical strategies extension together.

Social health insurance is a crucial component of integrated social protection strategies. Coverage extension through social insurance is possible and actions must be taken, in the short-term a pluralistic approach seems most promising, and these approaches should not lose sight of the long-term goal of adequate protection through social insurance. Existing social security institutions administering social health insurance schemes have a key role in promoting coverage within integrated strategies.

7.4 Health Care Financing and Provider Payment System

7.4.1 Framework to Improve Health Care Financing Arrangement

The framework consist of three aspects: generation, pooling, payment. The chief goal of improving health care financing arrangement is ensuring adequate and sustainable amount of resources to health care and reducing OOP health expenditure, removing financial barriers to care, and reducing catastrophic effect and impoverishment due to illness at the same time. The third goal is improving efficiency and effectiveness of health care financing.

7.4.2 Conceptual Framework for Provider Payment Systems

The conceptual framework consists of the following aspects: how to pay provider, kinds of payment. The unit of payment can be divided into five sections: service, case, time period, procedure, episode. And there are mainly four kinds of payment: fee-for-service (FFS) payment, DRG(Diagnosis Related Group)-based payment, capitation and budgeting.

Similar to the role of copayment in health insurance, balance between financial risk and incentives should be kept. If we take full protection against financial risk, there will be no incentive to reduce medical costs and leading to over-provision, over-utilization and inefficiency. In the other extreme, if we take no protection for financial risk, providers are 100% responsible for costs greater than payment, there will be strong incentive to reduce cost, but problems of access to care occur more frequently in health service.

The quality of care is another fact that we can not lose sight of. Providers paid by bigger units of payment have incentives to reduce quality, not to admit patients, or to admit less-severe cases. At the same time, providers have incentives to keep patients healthy, e.g., under capitation payment (then patient's utilization of medical care declines, which means savings and profits to providers), but it has potentials of leading to under-provision of care. Providers paid by fee-for-service have incentives to provide more services, admit more patients, or are neutral in terms of the severity of patients. This type of payment has no negative impact on access. However, owning to lacking of incentive to keep the fee of services, it will possibly lead to over-provision. Capitation/budgeting [fee-for-service] payment suffers from quality problem associated with under [over]-provision of services. Effect of different types of payment system on quality based on patient outcomes is not clear.

The amount of payment will produce effect on quality and access. If the level of payment to health care providers is too low, patients may have to pay informal payment.

7.4.3 Two main ways of payment

7.4.3.1 Fee-for-Service Payment

Fee-for-service (FFS) is a payment model where services are unbundled and paid for separately. In health care, it gives an incentive for physicians to provide more treatments because payment is dependent on the quantity of care, rather than quality of care. It raises costs, discourages the efficiencies of integrated care, and a variety of reform efforts have been attempted, recommended, or initiated to reduce its influence (such as moving towards bundled payments and capitation). It's difficult to set the fee level or judge the adequacy of fee level. Because reported cost or reported financial status (performance) of hospitals may be misleading, providers tend not to report true cost. Even with true reporting, it may not be based on efficient/optimal practice of providers. Industry attractiveness is a better indicator for the adequacy of fee level: entry of physicians (admission to medical schools) and private hospitals continues if the fee (measure of profitability) is reasonable.

To overcome the problems, it's necessary to take negotiation on the conversion factor.

In the past, a uniform conversion factor was applied to medical care, dental care, and traditional medical care, Recently, separate negotiation on conversion factors for different types of health care (medical doctors, dentists, traditional medical doctors).

7.4.3.2 DRG-based Payment System

Diagnosis-related group (DRG) is a system to classify hospital cases into one of originally 467 groups, with the last group (coded as 470 through v24, 999 thereafter) being "Ungroupable". This system of classification was developed as a collaborative project by Robert B. Fetter, PhD, of the Yale School of Management, and John D. Thompson, MPH, of the Yale School of Public Health. The system is also referred to as "the DRGs", and its intent was to identify the "products" that a hospital provides. In this payment, each patient is assigned to

DRG codes, payment for DRGs is fixed regardless of actual cost or length of stay. Payment is usually based on national mean, but can be adjusted to extreme cases (outliers) or provider type (e.g., high fee for tertiary care or teaching hospitals).

DRG is usually applied for inpatient care because it is easier to define the case (episode of care) than in outpatient care. Case-based payment has great impact on the health services. First it will lead to cost containment and decline in LOS (length of stay), and substitute unregulated care (e.g., outpatient, home health care) for regulated care (inpatient). The health providers tend to select lower-severity patients in a given case. Also, the implementation of this payment needs monitoring potential side-effects and the support of information system.

DRG and budget-based payment system has far-reaching impact on the quality of care. If the customary level of care is too high as a result of overprovision, then the reduction in quantity does not affect patient outcome negatively. If the customary level of care is optimal, a reduction in quantity leads to low quality and worse outcomes of patients.

In a matter of costing issues, it is hard to assess the true (justifiable) cost, providers have no incentive to be efficient, even if providers report true cost, it is too high if it is a result of inefficient practice style. And there are lots of evidence on inefficiency in physician practice. Moreover, implementing a sophisticated costing system for DRG (or fee setting in the FFS) can be too costly, costing (pricing) of individual services depends critically on the allocation of overhead (joint costs, e. g. electricity, salary of administrative personnel) to individual services.

The level of payment depends on the base rate, hospital type and outliers. For incremental implementation, one can use the mix of nation-wide and hospital-specific base rate at the beginning of the implementation. But the adjustment for the hospital-specific base rate is rewarding the high-cost hospitals, which can be caused by inefficiency or high severity of patients. Facility-specific base rate is not recommended also because it is difficult to abolish it later. A better option is to use nation-wide base rate, not facility-specific rate, to provide incentives for hospitals to improve efficiency. Base rate can be determined by top-down process (rather than bottom-up approach of costing), considering budget constraint or its impact on overall health insurance expenditure. Higher pay for tertiary care can accommodate the higher investment cost of tertiary care hospitals, but may induce over-investment in those hospitals. Same payment to primary, secondary and tertiary care hospitals for the same case, patients may prefer tertiary care if they perceive the quality of care in tertiary care hospitals is better . When it comes to the outliers, there are two different views on it. The pros held that the outliers reduce the perverse incentive of hospitals for patient selection or dumping, while the cons think that it can be abused by providers and can reduce provider incentives to minimize costs.

7.5   Case Study

Disparities in reimbursement for TB care among the three health insurance schemes in Yichang, China.

7.5.1   Population: Who Is Covered?

The three health insurance schemes have coverage of over 95% of the total population in all three counties. All three schemes offer inpatient and outpatient reimbursement for TB care in different forms.

The NCMS emphasizes coverage of TB inpatient services and hospitalization expenditures can be reimbursed with some co-payment. There are three modes of outpatient reimbursement as part of the NCMS: (1) household savings accounts, which can be used by beneficiaries directly to pay for outpatient expenditures; (2) outpatient reimbursement, which reimburses outpatient fees up to a certain amount at county and/or township level; (3) outpatient reimbursement for selected catastrophic or chronic illnesses, which compensates for large outpatient expenditures by establishing a catastrophic or chronic illness pooling fund. This includes diseases that are expensive to treat, but don't necessarily require admission to hospital (e. g. nephropathy, hepatitis, diabetes, hypertension). All three counties adopt this three-level structure.

Reimbursements for TB outpatient care are available at township, village, or community health facilities. Tuberculosis patients who have to seek treatment in the county-level TB designated hospitals cannot claim reimbursement for general outpatient care. Because of this, the NCMS provides a package covering chronic diseases, including TB, which means that TB patients can claim reimbursement for outpatient care accordingly.

The UEBMI consists of a pooled fund for inpatient stays and individual medical savings accounts for outpatient visits. In terms of TB care, the UEBMI offers inpatient and outpatient reimbursement for chronic diseases (a similar structure to the NCMS).

The URBMI seeks to eliminate impoverishment caused by high medical expenses by focusing on inpatient and outpatient services for chronic and fatal diseases, such as diabetes and heart disease. Tuberculosis patients are not covered by a package covering services for chronic diseases, however, they can still claim for inpatient and general outpatient reimbursement.

7.5.2   Services: Which Services Are Covered?

The NCMS offers a narrower benefit package than the other two schemes. Eleven anti-TB drugs are included in the NCMS, namely streptomycin, isoniazid, rifampicin, ethambutol, aminosalicylate sodium, pyrazinamide, rifapentine, and rifamycin, among others, whereas 20 drugs are covered by the UEBMI and the URBMI. Drugs are estimated to account for just under half of TB patient's OOP expenses. A more inclusive drug reimbursement list could help reduce

TB patients' OOP expenses by decreasing non-reimbursable expenses. According to our data results related to TB inpatients, non-reimbursable expenses rates for those covered by the NCMS from 2010 to 2012 in YD, ZJ, and WF were 7.8%, 13.34%, and 5.8%, respectively.

7.5.3 Costs: Proportion of the Costs Covered

The ability of health insurance schemes to reduce the financial burden of patients depends on the amount of funds that can be raised and pooled. Compared to the UEBMI, the URBMI and the NCMS have low financing. In YC city, for the NCMS, the annual premium per person was RMB 290 in 2012; for the URBMI, it was RMB 200; and for the UEBMI, it was usually over RMB 1000. Thus, the NCMS and URBMI have very basic benefit packages, which means they don't provide their beneficiaries with adequate funds to alleviate the economic hardships caused by serious diseases.

Tuberculosis patients who are covered by the UEBMI enjoy a more generous inpatient reimbursement policy. In this scheme, overall reimbursement rates increase with medical expenses rather than being determined by the level of the medical institution/hospital where the patient sought treatment. The ceiling is four times that of the average wage in the locality.

The NCMS reimbursement rates are higher than those of the URBMI, but lower than those of the UEBMI. Reimbursement for TB inpatient services is the same as for other inpatient services covered by the NCMS. The higher the level of the medical institution in which a patient receives treatment, the more he/she needs to pay out of pocket. The ceiling level for reimbursement ranged from RMB 100000 to RMB 150000.

Chapter 8　Hospital Information System

An electronic medical records (EMR) sharing platform is being developed in Beijing in 2015, which includes a national platform for EMR in China. Data, information and archives belong to 30 hospitals on this platform. What's more, 8 reginal platforms could be shared and inter-operated. Before that, if patients need their medical records or test results from the former hospitals when they go to another hospital, they have to look for the former records at home or from the former hospitals. If they cannot find the former results, they have to do all the tests once again. Now both of the patients and hospitals are able to access EMR from this platform whenever and wherever they need on a computer. All of that need a base that is able to collect, store, provide and demonstrate all kinds of information in hospital, which one we call it hosptial information system (HIS).

8.1　Introduction

The development of information and communication technology (ICT) has affected the society in general and health care system in particular. The use of digital tools in health care is dramatically increasing, and new technologies such as mobile devices and multifunctional bedside terminals are proliferating either. Documentation efforts are continuously rising and lead to the rapid development of sophisticated computer-based documentation tools. Decision support tools, such as the context of prescription supports high-quality care. Communication is increasingly supported by electronic means.

Systematic processing of information contributes to high quality patient care and reduces costs. As we all know, HIS strongly influences quality and efficiency of health care, and technical progress offers advanced opportunities to support health care. We will discuss hospital information system on the following questions:

(1) What is the hospital information system ?

(2) What is the classification of hospital information system?

(3) What are the functions and structures of the hospital information system?

(4) What is the essencial part of hospital information system?

8.1.1　Hospital Information System

Hospital information system(HIS) is an information management system which covers the whole process of the hospital business. The recognized definition was by Morris F. Collen: Hospital information system have taken the advantages of computers and communication equipment for the department of hospital, and the HIS is based on the licensing platform which could provide information collection, storage, process and retrieve, besides, the platform can also get patients' care information and administration information and meet the functional requirements of the authorized users.

China's Ministry of Health Information Work Leading Group Office of the revision of the "hospital information system Basic Functional Specification" formally defined the HIS: Hospital information system refers to taking use of the means of modern computer hardware and software technology, network communication technology, integrating management of hospital and its affiliated departments of human flow, material flow and financial flow, which plays a role in the medical activities in various stages of data acquisition, storage, processing, extraction, transmission and collection, and producing each kind of information, so as to the overall operation of the hospital provides comprehensive and automation of management and service information system. Hospital information system is the indispensable infrastructure and supporting environment in the modernization hospital construction.

A hospital information system can be regarded as the memory and nerve system of a hospital. Information and communication technology has become economically important and decisive for the quality of health care. It will continue to change health care.

8.1.2 The Characteristics of Hospital Information System

The information system of the hospital is regarded as the most complex enterprise information system in the world which was determined by the objectives, tasks and the hospital itself. HIS not only need to track management with the management information flow, financial flow and logistics in order to improve the operation efficiency of the hospital, but also help to support patient medical record information as the center of the medical, scientific and research activities.

(1) The HIS is the core of the database. The network is an environment supported by technology, which has a certain scale of the computer system.

(2) The HIS is the main line of business which can improve the quality and efficiency of work and decision-making. The main purpose is to improve the comprehensive management, reflect the panorama of enterprises, enhance the enterprise competition and get more and better social and economy benefits from the information system.

(3) Within the system, according to certain principles which are divided into several subsystems, each subsystem and system between mutual interface can effectively exchange information, which can make the sharing of true information come into realization.

(4) It has structured data, semi-structured data or unstructured data. Some data and architecture will be dramatically influenced by artificial intervention and social factors no matter

if they are static or dynamic.

(5) The HIS has perfect management, supervision and security system, and the corresponding rules, regulations and system security measures.

However, the hospital information system also has many different characteristics from the unique characteristics of general MIS. These characteristics tend to its own special design and bring greater difficulties.

(1) In many cases, it requires extremely rapid responses and online transaction processing capability. When an emergency patient is admitted to hospital, his timely and accurate medical records is of great importance for diagnosis. At the daily peak time, therapeutic-hall is crowded with hundreds of patients and their families, who queue anxiously when registrating, waiting, pricing, and taking medicine. The OLTP system's requirements are said to be no less than any bank window business system, air ticket booking and sales system.

(2) The complexity of medical information. Patients' information is expressed in a variety of data types, which contains text, data, graphics, images and so on.

(3) The requirements of information security and confidentiality. The patient's medical record is a file with the force of law. It works not only in the cases of medical disputes, but in many other legal processes, it will play an important role. The patient's information has a strict confidentiality requirements about charges, drugs, medical treatments and so on.

(4) The big data. The patient's medical records are growing faster and faster. It is common that a large hospital has millions of copies of the patient records.

(5) The lack of medical information processing standards. This is another outstanding problem to the development of complex hospital information system. At present, there are a few standards of medical information and information system for hospital management. Computer professionals in the information systems development process have spent great energy to deal with the field of information standardization that they are not familiar with, and participate in the formulation of some hospital management model and algorithm. The standardization of medical knowledge expression is how to translate medical knowledge into the form of a computer. We cannot realize the realistic electronic medical records without the problem being resolved.

(6) The overall goal of the hospital system, organization, management method, information flow model uncertainty, which increased the difficulties of analysis, design and implementation.

(7) A high demand of information sharing: the extent of medical knowledge of a doctor (e.g. a new drug usage and dosage, the taboo, a kind of special cases described in the literature and the conclusions) and patient medical records (both in the demand for hospital patients or several years before the death of the patients) may occur in all his medicine, teaching and research activities. And an inpatient hospitalization records abstract (the first page of the medical record) may also be required from the clinical departments of a hospital, medical

departments and the administrative department (from the guard until dean). So the design of HIS must ensure that the speed and safety of information transmission or sharing and the reliability of the network.

(8) The management of medical staff psychological and behavioral disorders. The success of the hospital information system depends on hospital medical staff and administrators involved. The psychological and behavioral obstacles of medical staff and administrators often lead to a systematic failure. In China, due to the universal education background, the popularization of computer and the difficulty of Chinese characters input, so the end user is more general and strong to resist the use of computer. This requires that the system designers pay more attention to the interface of human friendly design, and help to make it more convenient to learn the information and simple operation, and efficient character information input. Of course, that in turn increases the overhead and complexity of the system.

8.1.3 Functions and Significance of Hospital Information System

8.1.3.1 Functions

According to the functional attribution and the characteristics of hospital, the hospital information system should have the following basic functions:

(1) Collect and permanently store all data required for the hospital. Because of the complexity of hospital information, especially the information of the patient with the characteristics of the dynamic data structure, the hospital information system should have the capacity of big storage.

(2) Data sharing. It is to provide the hospital with the necessary data and support the basic activities of the hospital operation.

(3) A function of individual transaction processing, comprehensive transaction processing and assistant decision-making.

(4) The effective function of data management and data communication is to ensure data accurate, reliable, confidential and secure.

(5) In order to ensure the medical activities and hospital running uninterrupted, the system should have the function of continuous operation.

(6) Effectively ensure the safety of the system.

(7) The necessary softwares and databases for the developing research of the system.

(8) A good user environment. The end user's application and operation should be simple, convenient, easy to learn and easy to understand.

(9) The system is scalable. Hospital information system is an important tool and means of the modern hospital management. It is an important guarantee for the deepening of hospital reformation, refining management, improving efficiency and extending the information service, and it has great significance to improve competitiveness. Such as optimizing workflow, which is able to improve operation quality, shorten the diagnosis and treatment cycle, strengthen scientific management, save the costs of diagnosis and treatment, and change decision-making mode.

8.1.3.2　Significance

The health information system has changed health care which is not only important for economy but also decisive for the quality of health care. We will talk about the significance of HIS according to its impact on quality of care and economics, and changing the way of health care.

(1) Improving the quality of health care. Information system can change the costs and quality of information processing in health care. The role of computer-supported information systems, together with clinical documentation and knowledge-based decision support systems can hardly be overestimated in respect to the quality of health care, as the volume of data available today is much greater than it was a few years ago.

(2) Increasing economics. HIS in health care also emerged to a leading industry branch. There is a significant and increasing economical relevance for information and communication technology in general but also in health care.

(3) Improving health care. Computer-based information systems strongly support efficient learning for doctors. With the help of HIS, documentations about patient health are continuous and convenient. Decision support systems, for example, in the context of drug prescription, support high-quality care. Communication is increasingly supported by electronic.

Information processing is not conducted globally across institutions, but locally. This corresponds to traditional separation politics and leads to isolated information processing groups, such as the administration or the clinic.

In short, through the implementation of hospital information system, we can infer it is able to effectively promote the construction of hospital information and management of hospital; help to integrate employees to work more efficiently, simple relations of department cooperation; reveal the department revenue and expenses of patients with list, electronic information of diagnosis and treatment; efficiently and orderly standardize medical service process; bring new environment of diagnosis and treatment to the hospital and patients, and provide better medical services.

8.1.4　Structure and Model of Hospital Information System

The structure of the hospital information system is directly related to the medical activity. The structure of hospital information system is as follows:

(1) The clinical part: doctor workstation, nurse workstation, clinical laboratory information system, medical imaging system, blood transfusion and blood bank management system, anesthesia management system and so on.

(2) The Drug adminstration part: (data preparation and drug dictionary, drug warehouse management, outpatient pharmacy management, pharmacy management, drug charge, drug price management, preparation management subsystem, the rational use of drugs advisory function.

(3) Economic management: outpatient registration system, delimiting price system in emergency, inpatients and outpatient, charge system, material management system, equipment management subsystem, financial and accounting management system.

(4) Comprehensive management and statistical analysis: medical record management system, medical statistics system, inquiry and analysis system, and consultation service system for patients.

(5) External interface: medical insurance interface, community health service interface, remote medical consultation system interface.

The composition of the hospital information system consists of two parts: the hardware systems and the software systems. The hardware systems have high performance of center computer or server, and device of large storage, throughout the hospital departments of the user terminal equipment and data communication circuit, composed of information resource sharing computer network. The computer software systems are oriented to multiple users and multiple functions, including system software, application software and software development tools, various hospital information database and database management system.

From the system function and subdivision, hospital information system generally can be divided into three parts: first is to meet the management requirements of the management information system; second is to meet the medical requirements for medical information system; third is to meet the two requirements of information service system above, and the systems can be divided into several subsystems. In addition, many hospitals also undertake clinical teaching and research, social health care, medical insurance and other tasks, so the hospital information system should also be set up to the corresponding information system.

(1) The architectures of hospital information system is complicated and specific. The function and the way of implementation of the subsystems are varied. But from the view of the system theory and information theory, the entity data structure and abstraction concept of information processing of the hospital information system can be used a simple model to describe the basic composition.

(2) The model of hospital information system consists of 6 levels: the first level is the user, according to the actual users to design HIS; the second level is the user terminal, based on the users' activity applications given the terminal different functions (such as computers, multimedia computer graphics workstations, etc.); the third level called application environment, which is the hospital information system hardware and software, providing application device of the mixture for the user, such as window operation, screen, keyboard function keys, printing tools, auxiliary equipment, etc.; the fourth level is the application of

hospital information system and subsystem. In this level, the user can enter the hospital information system to complete the relevant functions; the fifth level is data base management system(DBMS), under the level of the database requirements, which all applications can communicate with the DBMS and access database, all data in the database can also be accessed and shared all applications by in accordance with the requirements; the sixth level is the real database, storing various types of data about hospital management and patient diagnosis and treatment. These data obtained from users applications and the DBMS. The Table 8-1 is architectures of hospital information system.

Table 8-1 **Hospital Information System Architectures**

the sixth level: database
the fifth level: database management system
the fourth level: hospital information system
the third level: application environment
the second level: user terminal
the first level: user

8.1.5 Current Hospital Information System in China

Nearly all people and all areas of hospitals are affected by the quality of the information system, as most of them need various types of information in their daily work. The patient certainly profit most from high-quality information processing since it contributes to the quality of patient care and to reducing costs. The professional groups working in a hospital, especially physicians, nurses, and administrative personnel, are also directly affected by the quality of the information system.

(Information processing has to integrate the partly overlapping information of the different groups and areas of a hospital.) Systematic and integrated information processing in the hospital have advantages not only for the patient, but also for the health care professionals, the health insuance companies and the hospital's owners. Systematic processing of information contributes to high quality patient care and reduced costs. The integrated processing of information is important, because all groups of people and all areas of hospitals depend on its quality, the amount of information processing in hospitals is considerable, and health care professionals frequently work with the same data.

In China, after 30 years of development, the hospital or software company has invested a lot of manpower, material and financial resources to improve hospital information system. County hospitals have built their own hospital management information system basically, and the developed township hospital is also starting to build their own hospital management information system. These phenomena are fully described, the construction of hospital information system have stepped in a new level and everybody understands the importance and necessity of hospital information system construction.

In 2001, the Ministry of Health Statistics showed that the majority of provincial affiliated hospital have been built HIS, above 38% of county-level hospitals applied information technology.

In 2005, the hospital management professional members surveyed of 482 hospital in China on the hospital management information system online. Survey showed that all the systems, such as HMIS, charging information system, emergency system and outpatient prescriptions, admission discharge hospital management information system, cost management information system, inpatient pharmacy management information system and storeroom management information system had the advantage of lowing down cost. And all the system construction condition was good, above 90% of the systems are on-line.

In 2007, Ministry of Health Statistical Information Center surveyed nationwide of 3765 hospitals, the survey showed that the outpatient charges information system, outpatient pharmacy management information system, hospitals patient cost management information system and the drug storehouse management system were most widely used. The charge system were the center of HMIS and more than 80% of hospitals applied it. Patient referral management information system, inpatient bed management information system, hospital pharmacy management information system were used in more than 70% hospitals.

According to the report of Chinese hospital information status investigation of 2012—2013, in nationwide, 1067 hospitals clinical information system implementation status were surveyed. The results showed that: in more than 70% of hospitals, the nurses station system, hospital doctor workstation system, outpatient doctor workstation system, electronic medical records system were the most widely used and had been implemented or were prepared to implement; in more than 60% of hospitals, the laboratory information system, picture archiving and communication system (PACS) and ultrasound imaging information system had been implemented or were ready for implementation; more than 50% of hospitals, the medical center management system, radiology information system and internal peep mirror imaging system had been implemented or were ready for implementation. The degree of hospital health information system is increasing, especially the electronic medical record system.

8.2　Hospital Management Information System

Hospital information system (HIS) should include both the hospital management information system(HMIS) and the clinical medical information system(CMIS). The main goal of the HMIS is to support the hospital administration management and transaction processing business, to mitigate the labor intensity of the workers, to assist hospital management and senior leadership decision-making and improve hospital efficiency, thus it enables the hospital to obtain the better social benefit and economic benefit with less investment. Financial system, personnel system, hospital patient management system, drug inventory management system belong to HMIS.

CMIS is including medical expert system, auxiliary diagnosis system, auxiliary teaching system, monitoring system for critical patients, drug counseling and monitoring system, and some special medical systems, such as CT (computer X-ray tomography), ultrasound, ECG automatic analysis, blood cells and automatic biochemical analysis. Information system directly relates to hospital management activities. The system is relatively independent, and forms a special system, and is controlled by the special computer, mainly to complete data acquisition and preliminary analysis, exchange integrated medical documents and medical database, query and call the doctor and so on, the results of which can be acquired through the network.

The function of hospital information management system is mainly the economic management, medicine management, clinical diagnosis and treatment, comprehensive management and statistical analysis, external interface.

8.2.1　Economic Management

Economy is the lifeblood of the hospital, and it is the basis of the doctor's survival and development. The goal of economic management is rationally used in hospital resources and efficient organization of medical treatment, teaching, scientific research work and improving the quality of hospital care, medical effect and economic effect. It mainly includes:

8.2.1.1　Outpatient Management

(1) Registered system. It support a variety of registration form, automatic generation number table, provide inquiries, statistical functions, for the follow-up medical information. It can quickly establish the patient identification code and reduce the waiting time of the patients in the treatment process. For example, patient admission aims at recording and distributing the patient demographics and insurance data as well as medical and nursing data of the patient history. In addition, each patient must be correctly identified, a unique patient and case identifier must be assigned.

(2) Charge subsystem. The system providing pricing, fees, refund, print reimbursement vouchers, settle accounts, statistics, query and other services. Charges integration improves work efficiency and service quality, and reduces the work intensity. And the main goal of the system is optimizing the financial supervision system.

8.2.1.2　Hospital Management

Management is the center of the hospital work, and it reflects the service quality of hospital.

（1）Patient admission and outpatient system. Admission is the first step in medical services, access to patient information and placement of patients. Standardizing the scientific admission process can effectively reduce medical errors, avoid disputes. Hospital discharge process reflects the collaborative work ability of each department in hospital, and also the connecting point of all kinds of hospitals. The information transfer is the focus of hospital management.

（2）Inpatient charge subsystem. There are many difficulties in the hospital management, such as high cost of hospitalization, complexity of information process, all kinds of participation and the duration of the management. Charge subsystem, combined with the decentralized mode and the traditional mode, can maximally avoid leakage fee. The decentralized mode is reflected in the two aspects of pricing and charging. The fees of patients are produced in the decentralized pricing information system. For example, in costs unit, doctor workstations subsystem and nurse workstation's system respectively take charge of costs independent generated in the image, inspection department, medical imaging subsystem and clinical test subsystem.

（3）Facility management subsystem. The hospital equipment and logistics material are the basic condition for the orderly development of the medical, teaching and scientific research in the hospital. The mobility and randomness of the business object of the hospital expand the demand for the logistics material in hospital. Information system realizes scientific management of the entire life cycle of the hospital equipment and logistics, cost accounting management and provide data base for decision-making, optimize the allocation of resources, control the loss of property. It is including hospital purchase management, inventory management, maintenance management, and depreciation management. (The Figure 8-1 shows the enterprise function facility management.)

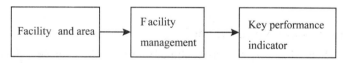

Figure 8-1   The Enterprise Function Facility Management, Its Subfunctions and Interpreted and Updated Entity Types

（4）Financial accounting management subsystem. Financial management is based on hospital development in the process of financial activities information, including budget management, revenue management, expenditure and cost management, balance and distribution, debt management, financial settlement, from the financial reporting and analysis. The economic management subsystem is used for the hospital economic accounting and department accounting, including the hospital income and expenditure, the department's income and expenditure, the cost of the hospital and the department. The Figure 8-2 shows enterprise function financial management.

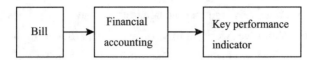

Figure 8-2   The Enterprise Function Financial Management, Its Subfunctions and
Interpreted and Updated Entity Types

8.2.2   Drug Management

Drug is a substance administered to a patient for treatment diagnosis or prevention. Drug management system assists the entire hospital to complete the management of drugs, deals with medical and pharmaceutical activities of relevant data, drug storage, preparation, outpatient pharmacy, hospital pharmacy, drug prices, drug accounting information management and assists the rational use of drugs. The main functions include:

8.2.2.1   Drug Dictionary Management

The standard drug dictionary includes a rich set of attributes: code category, name, dosage form, classification of toxicology, classification of prescription, medical insurance category, taking methods, use restrictions, manufacturers, suppliers, packaging, specifications, price, etc. Through the definition of key attributes, user (medical personnel) can accurately locate the only one drug, that is the basic requirements of drug data dictionary. Drug dictionary can provide comprehensive and accurate information about the drug for hospital information system and medical personnel. And drug dictionary can avoid confusion and reduce error rate of pharmaceutical activities.

8.2.2.2   Pharmacy Store Management

Pharmacy store is the hospital concentrated reserve drug place which dispatches the medicine from the pharmacy to meet the daily needs of the hospital. Take the drug dictionary as the template, the pharmacy store automatically or artificially collects the basic information of the medicine and stores it in the database. When outpatient pharmacy and inpatient pharmacy extract drug information from the database, they can regularly change the status of drug, and then feedback to the pharmacy store. Figure 8-3 is about pharmacy store process.

8.2.2.3   Pharmacy Accounting Management

Pharmacy accounting management bases on cost and benefit as the main index, includs the hospital drug circulation and medicine, scientific pharmaceutical activities, comprehensive statistics, accounting and analysis. It starts from the two dimensions of hospital or department,

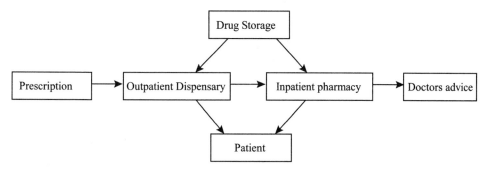

Figure 8-3 Pharmacy store process

increased the planning and combined with local control. The main functions of pharmacy accounting management are:

(1) Automatic and manual provide uniform adjustment of hospital drug price function, and record the relevant information, such as price adjustment details, time, cause and the profit and loss.

(2) Sharing the financial management subsystem data, provide automatic and manual reimbursement function.

(3) Pharmacy accounting management provide financial processing and statistical analysis functions, such as checking import and storeroom, pharmacy prescription, drug receipts and so on, regular statistical analysis of hospital medicine and pharmacy, pharmacy operating costs and benefits.

(4) Hospital pharmacy consumption activity statistics.

(5) Output under a unified format and content, just like output the generation of accounting books to output pharmacy report.

The pharmacy costs and benefits are important parts of hospital economy. Pharmacy finance management information system can be effectively control the cost of pharmacy, reduce the loss of the drug, and improve pharmacy service quality and patients' satisfaction.

8.2.2.4 Preparation Management

The preparation management is a variety of specific application of drugs, biological and other drugs, such as drugs, biology, etc., according to pharmacopoeia or drug standards, preparation management provides effective function to meet the needs of treatment or prevention. It's the important supplement to the development of the pharmaceutical market and the hospital economy.

(1) Warehouse management, including raw materials, packaging materials storage, out of the warehouse, inventory, sales and other management.

(2) Procurement management, such as planning, procurement, payment and payment management.

(3) Semi-finished and finished product management.

(4) Accounting management.

(5) Quality control, such as finished inspection, etc.

(6) Production process management.

(7) Output documents, vouchers and statements.

8.2.2.5 Rational Drug Use Consultation

(1) The potential irrational drug use review and warning function in the prescription or medical order.

(2) Drug information inquiry function.

(3) Brief medication reminder function.

The working principle of rational drug use consultation is the special value of judging and recognizing the attribute of drug dictionary and the corresponding result. It contributes to improving the quality of pharmaceutical service, reducing the mistake of prescription and medicine.

8.2.3 Human Resources Management

Human resources(HR) refers to the certain period of the hospital needs of these people to meet the needs of the human resources. As a special economic and social resource, man is the backbone of hospital running. Human resource management system functions as following:

(1) Human resources planning;

(2) Recruitment and allocation staffs;

(3) Training and development staffs;

(4) Remuneration and benefits management;

(5) Performance management;

(6) Employee relationship management;

(7) Personnel management;

(8) Career management;

(9) Self-service.

These functions are interrelated and interacted with each other, which constitute the whole process of human resource management. Performance management is the core of human resource management subsystem.

8.2.4 Comprehensive Management and Statistical Analysis

The function of this is about statistical analysis and management for all kinds of related data of hospital, and all of the data gathering, analysis, comprehensive treatment for leadership decision-making and medical statistics.

8.2.4.1 Medical Statistics Subsystem

The function of medical statistics subsystem is collection, storage, statistical analysis and providing accurate data of hospital development, utilization of resources, medical care quality, medical departments work efficiency for hospitals and health management departments to provide a variety of reports. The abnormal report has a high reference value in the hospital for epidemic prediction and market evaluation.

8.2.4.2 Comprehensive Query and Analysis Subsystem

Comprehensive query and analysis subsystem is the supervisor support system providing data query and analysis for the hospital leadership to master the hospital operation status. It is from hospital management information system in price with the hospital management of medical treatment, teaching, scientific research and decision-making information analysis and detection of possible strategic opportunities and threats.

8.2.4.3 Patient Counseling Subsystem

The main task of patient counseling subsystem is providing medical guidances and the consulting services to patients by telephone, Internet, touch screen, etc.

8.2.5 External Interface

This function provides the interface of the hospital information system and the new rural cooperative medical system. We progressively realize the interface of the medical insurance system, two-way system of diagnosis and treatment, and remote medical consultation system, maternal and child health care system. And external interface can solve the interconnection problems of hospital and social system.

8.2.5.1 Medical Insurance Interface

Medical insurance interface is used to help complete the information exchange between the image system and the higher medical insurance department. The main task is to help hospitals in accordance with the national medical insurance policy for medical insurance patients to solve a variety of cost settlement processing.

8.2.5.2 Regional Health Service Interface

Regional health service interface provides a unified standard which is set for different data formats. The main task is to track the patients after discharge, improve service quality, provide fast and convenient service for patient referral. Regional health service interface is the premise and foundation of constructing regional health service system, and the medical data is concentrated and accurated for statistics and analysis, which is conducive to the health institution of disease prevention and control capacity.

8.2.5.3　Tel-medical System

Tel-medical system is the effective way to integrate medical resources and narrow the medical gap between difference regions of the economic development. The tel-medical system provides no difference and a high level of medical and health services to patients in different regions, and reduces the burden of patients, establishes a good relationship between doctors and patients. Hospital can also provide direct guidance language assistance for remote medical institutions, reduce medical costs, optimize the allocation of resources, strengthen exchanges and cooperation.

8.3　Clinical Information System

8.3.1　Introduction

The main goal of clinical information system(CIS) is to support the clinical activity of hospital medical staff. For example, CIS can collect and process the patient's clinical information, enrich and accumulate the knowledge of clinical medicine and provide clinical consultation, auxiliary diagnosis and treatment, clinical decision-making, improve the working efficiency of the medical staff, provide much faster and better services for patients. It includes the doctor order processing system, the patient bedside system, the doctor workstation system, the laboratory system, the medicine consultation system and so on.

The clinical information system has two different concepts compared to the hospital management information system. HMIS is a management system which mainly deals with the information of human, financial and material, etc.. It is geared to the needs of the hospital management. CIS is the management system that is based on the clinical information. Patients oriented CIS can serve the hospital staff and improve the quality of medical care.

8.3.2　Doctor Workstation System

It is for management of patient information, doctor information, diagnosis and treatment information and service for doctors quickly acquiring and processing information. The doctor workstation system has the following features:

(1) Standard medical records and medical advice writing. The doctor workstation system provides a standard template for doctors to record detailed and accurate patients information. Doctors use the mouse, keyboard, handwriting board or other input tools to fill in the data, which not only improve the efficiency of data entry, but also guarantee the quality of the document. At the same time, the system allows the standard template to add a custom field to meet the needs of the special medical event recorded. And the system has a high degree of

flexibility.

(2) Efficient information query is based on information sharing. Doctor workstation system provides the necessary information support for doctors to complete medical activities. Except supporting the basic information of patients, as well as the prescription, medical advice, inspection and other information, the system also provides a powerful medical record retrieval functions. This information comes from various information systems used in hospitals. Information sharing between the system is expanding the range of width and depth about query and retrieval. The emergence of new technologies such as data warehouse, online analysis and data mining, provides a new way for information retrieval and query.

(3) Strict management. Doctor workstation system supports management authority and makes accurate expression of the doctor's department. And it provides a reliable basis to strengthen the medical advice or medical records. The doctors workstation is divided into two parts, which are out-patient doctor workstation subsystem and resident doctor workstation subsystem.

The main function include:

(1) Dynamic generation about waiting patient information.

(2) Provide the auxiliary diagnosis and analysis for the doctor.

(3) Check the patient. The system has a complete laboratory inspection library, and provides a note of the examination items according to the doctor's needs.

(4) Give the patient a prescription and injection. Systems have built-in prescription generator function which is simple and easy to use. And this system contains western medicine library, Chinese medicine library, Chinese herbal medicine library which can provide instruction about drug attribute incompatibility according to the needs of physicians of drug administration.

(5) Generate medical records for the patients. Built-in system with electronic medical record can provide western medicine subjects according to the standards, which makes it convenient for doctors to entry medical record.

(6) Definition of commonly used prescription template for doctors' personal use.

(7) Use of a template definition utility of physician prescription.

(8) Doctors commonly used medical records management. According to the definition of the disease, the doctor can define the prescription, the optional prescription and the template of the outpatient medical record.

(9) Outpatient service includes patient archives information inquiry, complete prescription, expense, medical record, inspection result, inspection report, image report.

(10) Outpatient medical records statistical analysis table, according to the hospital's need for custom statistics.

Doctors workstation system not only reflects the service concept of the patient as the work center, but also helps doctors quickly improve service quality and work efficiency of diagnosis and treatment. The system would help doctors when they met the diseases which are difficult to diagnose and miscellaneous. Networking can also allow outpatient doctors rapidly get results feedback of test, imaging, and so on.

8.3.3   Nurse Workstation System

8.3.3.1   Features of the System

The system assists the ward nurse to complete the daily nursing work, and check and handle the long and temporary doctor's orders issued by him at the same time, and manages the execution of the doctor's orders.

(1) Facing clinical nursing, you should realize and understand the whole process management of the doctor's orders, and the standard of the doctor's orders.

(2) System can be convenient for patient's bed management of bulk billing, medical order management (entry, audit, void, stop and execution), executive management of inpatient and inspection reports and other daily management, powerful query capabilities.

(3) Easy input and friendly interface. The daily operation of the nurse can not enter any of the characters to complete the patient's and doctor's advices to work, in accordance with the nurse's advice processing input mode.

(4) System supports group orders, mutual exclusion orders, such as a variety of complex relations within a prescribed and intelligent to help nurses, improves the quality and efficiency of nursing.

(5) Being integrated with the doctors workstation, inspection and operation anesthesia, and so on.

8.3.3.2   Main Function

(1) Graphical display ward beds, enable the patient's bed number, hospital number, name, sex, illness, nursing grades and other information to be seen clearly, select patients after the details of synchronous display.

(2) Automatically receive the doctor orders. Generate the doctor's orders and print a variety of documents after auditing, and carry out the relevant cost management at the same time.

With the combination of the center, it can realize the function of the inquiry, printing and checking of the transfusion. It also supports centralized configuration and the sending of liquid.

(3) Prescription dispensing. Simple drag can realize medication orders. It supports single prescription medicine, nursing station summary of drug, and system combination of drug to achieve your doctor put medicine and a variety of modes.

(4) Simple and quick charging mode, which can greatly improve working efficiency.

(5) Special patient management. The special management of the special patients, such as medical insurance patients and SARS patients.

(6) Information inquiry. It includes cost list of one day, cost and deposit query, and hospitalization history query, and convenient access to the patient's past medical records, past medical history, medication records, inspection reports, the current condition of the development, the results of a variety of inspection, etc..

(7) Learning guide. To obtain the relevant medical knowledge through conveniently, it provides the diagnosis and treatment routine, the medicine manual, the inspection handbook, the medical information resources for each disease retrieval.

8.3.4 Laboratory Information System

Referred to laboratory information system (LIS) , it is a network system which can realize the automation of the information of clinical inspection and test information management. Its main function is experimental instrument which will automatically generate reports and print them after analyzing the outgoing inspection data that tested out, and store them in the database through the network, making it convenient and timely for the doctor to acquire inspection result of the patient. In present's application, LIS has become an essential part of digital hospital management.

The advanced inspection information system should have important functions such as the two-way communication with the doctor orders, the bar code management, the financial automatic charge, the instrument control, and so on.

Software for processing laboratory information. LIS is composed of a variety of laboratory process modules, which can be selected and configured according to the actual situation of customers. Choosing a suitable laboratory information system is very important for the users, and often costs several months of research and planning. The installation and adjustment of the system also range from several weeks to a few months, and the laboratory research work has many kinds of laboratory information systems. Large-scale LIS includes almost all subject contents of laboratory studies, such as blood, biochemistry, immunology, blood bank, surgical pathology, anatomical pathology, online cell count, and microbiology.

LIS can achieve the following functions: customizing inspection items, patient login, receiving sample, recording results, generating reports, statistics of patients and physicians, network customized tests based on network, results of which will be sent to the customers by fax and email, generating medical inspection table, balancing the workload, medical insurance and the necessity of examination, delimiting price to generate public health reports, formulating management rules.

8.3.5 Picture Archiving and Communications Systems

The goal of picture archiving and communications systems (PACS) is to support all hospital internal activities on the image, the integration of medical equipment, image storage and distribution, important diagnosis and consultation in the digital image display, image archiving, and external information system.

Medical imaging system is used for collecting, processing, storing, transmitting and searching for all kinds of medical image information. The function of medical imaging system can be divided into two parts.

8.3.5.1   Image Processing Section

(1) Data receiving function. Receive and acquire Digital Imaging and Communications in Medicine(DICOM) and non-DICOM format image data, and convert the image data of the non DICOM image to DICOM standard data.

(2) Image processing functions. Display the relevant information of images, such as name, age, equipment type, etc.. Provide scaling, transfering image, reversing, rotating, filtering, playback and other functions.

(3) Measurement function. Provide the measurement of length, angle, area and other data, as well as labeling, annotation function.

(4) Preservation. Support storage with different formats, as well as the conversion into DICOM format.

(5) Management functions. Support the transmission of images between devices, and have access to patients' image reports in different periods, different equipment. Support DICOM print output, mass data storage, and migration management.

(6) Telemedicine. Remote transmitting and receiving of image data.

(7) Parameter setting function. Support users to customize the size of the text, amplification ratio and other parameters.

8.3.5.2   Report Management

(1) Appointment registration function.

(2) Triage. The information about patient, inspection, and the charge.

(3) Diagnostic report function. Generate inspection reports. Support for the doctor review. Support for typical case management.

(4) Template function. Users can easily and flexibly define templates, improve the speed of report generation.

(5) Query function. Support for a variety of query forms, such as name, image number, etc.

(6) Statistical functions. You can count the users' workload, outpatient amount, film volume and cost information.

8.3.5.3   Medical Imaging System

The hospital using the X-ray imaging system, X-ray computed tomography system (CT), magnetic resonance imaging (MRI), electrocardiogram information system, computer information systems, etc. All that belong to the category of medical imaging system.

8.3.6 Operation and Anesthesia Management System

Manage the operation and anesthesia of patients in the hospital, and do research about record and tracking of operation. The arrangement of hospital operation and anesthesia is a complicated process, which requires reasonable, effective and safe. Operation and anesthesia management can effectively ensure the normal operation of hospital.

According to the operation procedure, operation and anesthesia management system can be divided into the following functions.

8.3.6.1 Before Surgery

Provide basic information related of patients and surgery, according to the relevant provisions complete application and approval of the operation and anesthesia, complete arrangement of the operation, anesthesia personnel, supplies and equipment, confirm all ready before operation, record the preoperative consultation information, and discuss and summarize the information.

8.3.6.2 Operation

Provide basic information of patients related to surgical and anesthesia, and verification information involved operation of the doctors and nurses; automatically acquire patient's vital signs parameters, automatically generate log of operation and anesthesia operation, record surgery, anesthesia during the event detailedly; get access to electronic patient records and database in the history of medical record data ready, provide a reliable basis for decision making.

8.3.6.3 After Surgery

Automatically acquire, monitor the patient's vital signs parameters and record the postoperative follow-up information, complete the whole process of operation information summary and providing cost information; check records of operation and anesthesia, save , query, statistics and analysis the data.

Compared with the traditional process of anesthesia and operation, operation management system provides information that conforms to the standards and requirements of the disease according to the standardize data operation code database; read the patient vital signs data directly from the medical instruments and equipments, according to the anesthesia and operation activities automatically generate operation log, check the information before operation and after operation many times, improve the authenticity of the input and transmission relevant information in the process of operation system; strict division of authority, to ensure the validity and security of medical activities; for emergency, rescue and other special circumstances, simplify the arrangement of operation anesthesia procedures, allowing makeup after the operation related data shows, improve the flexibility of the system; realize data communication and sharing between operation and anesthesia management system and other system interface, creating favorable conditions for the improvement of medical treatment .

8.3.7   Medical Record Management Subsystem

Medical record is medical staff to record the process of disease diagnosis and treatment, it is objective, complete and continuous, recording of changes of the patient's diagnosis, treatment, the treatment effect and outcome. Medical record management subsystem is a system for the management of medical record and related work of medical record department. Medical record is the important data source of hospital medical education, scientific research which can provide reliable statistical results for medical workers to retrieval flexibly and conveniently, the main task of the system is to reduce the workload of the medical record management staff. Its management includes medical record home management, name index management, medical record lending, medical record, medical record quality control and patient follow up management.

Medical record management subsystem is the product of the information system of the hospital in the knowledge economy environment, and belongs to the knowledge management system. Medical record management subsystem will be recorded in the form of medical records in the database. Doctors can use fuzzy logic in the system to retrieve the similar characteristics of the history of medical records, to seek the best medical program.

8.3.8   Clinical Decision

Clinicians make full use of the system available, appropriate computer technology for semi-architecture or unarchitecture medical problems, through human-computer interaction which can improve the efficiency of decision-making .

When the patient's detailed data entered into the information system, it was stored in the database. Clinical decision support system locates and accesses data which is representative of the key information. After processing the information and then in the data model matching, thereby it generates a particular patient health assessment, diagnosis and treatment recommendations.

Decision support system provides a variety of methods to analyze and judge data in order to insure the quality of decision making. The general methods include Bayesian model, decision tree, artificial intelligence, neural network, and simulation model.

8.3.8.1   Bayesian Model

Practical diagnosis process is like this: according to what has been discovered and mastered by clinical manifestations, clinicians combine medical knowledge with experiences carries on the preliminary analysis and judgment, gradually do interrogation and examination, and then do further analysis and judgment, so as to keep the cycle until there is enough proof to make conclusions. Bayesian model is the information process, gradual and progressive analysis of the measurement and diagnosis. Bayesian model is to construct complete disease group firstly, and then determines the prior probability and conditional probability through a variety of known information, and establishes differential diagnosis of independent syndrome index, and then calculates the posterior probability. According to certain indicators, they screen and compare the results and come up the final conclusion.

8.3.8.2 Decision Tree

Decision tree is a kind of mathematical model, which is based on the tree effective expression of complex decision-making problem. The root node of the decision tree is the starting point of decision making. The decision maker judges the child nodes of the next layer on the basis of the specific criteria and begins a new round of selection. And then repeat this process until the decision tree is reached. Simply, the doctor in the diagnosis process, within the existing complex problem program, chooses "yes" or "no" , so as to complete the logic of the clinical decision-making process.

8.3.8.3 Artificial Intelligence

Artificial intelligence uses machine to simulate reasoning, learning and association. It is an important tool to simulate and extend the decision-making ability of people. In medical field, the research of artificial intelligence includes robot, language recognition, image recognition, natural language processing, and so on. Expert system is a typical product of the evolution of artificial intelligence, and it is the use of one or more experts providing medical domain knowledge using deductive logic or rules of thumb reasoning and judgment, which can solve the difficult problem of the medicine.

8.3.8.4 Neural Network

Neural network is a kind of behavior characteristic of simulating human or animal neural network, and the mathematical model of distributed parallel information processing is carried out by a large number of interconnected processing units. Neural network has the self learning and adaptive ability, analyzes and grasps the potential rules between the two from the input-output data, and uses the new input data to predict the output results.

8.3.8.5 Medical Simulation

Medical simulation model uses anatomy, kinesiology, biomechanics, geometry, computer science and other fields of professional knowledge, through computer modeling, collision detection, real-time computing, force feedback and other functions. The establishment of real tissues and organs of the human body is similar to the virtual model and simulation to various changes in the environment under the action of the tissues and organs of the human body and the operation personnel of sensory feedback. The characteristics of medical simulation model is direct, vivid and close to reality. It can be used to evaluate the value and risk of the medical personnel, and also can be used in medical record and so on.

8.4　Electronic Medical Record

8.4.1　What is Electronic Medical Record

The essence of hospital information is electronic medical record(EMR)

EMR is in electronic to record patient's information including home page, course records, inspection results, doctor's advice, surgical records, nursing records, all of which information in architecture and unarchitecture free text and graphics and image information, statistics and post processing of all recorded information and data in the treatment process. The acquisition, storage, transmission, quality control, statistics and utilization of patient's information. As the main source of information in medical treatment, the service exceeds the medical records and meets the needs of medical treatment, law and management.

The EMR is mainly created, used and saved by the medical institution, which is the main information source and important component of the health archives of the residents. Electronic medical record system writes records through the program and realizes the integration of medical information, sharing retrieval and monitoring etc. According to the country health department of the electronic medical record writing standard and maximum to follow the doctor's way of writing to design and greatly reduce the labor intensity of doctor in medical record writing.

The use of electronic medical record system, greatly improves work efficiency, save a lot of valuable time for medical personnel records, and extricate the medical staff from the heavy records task, so that medical personnel has more time for the observation of disease changes and patients' condition, better contact and communication with patients, and that patients get more care and better treatment. It is conducive to the establishment of a good relationship between doctors and patients, and at the same time, save more time for research and improve the medical skill. The use of the electronic medical record system also greatly improves the quality of the medical records, so that the medical records are more standardized and more valuable for research and utilization. Step to a new level of hospital management, monitoring and assessment of the department's work, the hospital management and assessment increase a means of management, medical records such as superior physician inspection and so on. The use of electronic medical records can speed up the circulation of patient information, and provides the medical records service for department that needs obtained the patient information. The use of the electronic medical record system has the advantages of achieving medical records to paperless, saves the hospital expenses, reduces operating costs and improves economic efficiency.

8.4.2　The Characteristics of Electronic Medical Records

(1) Transmission. Medical personnel can remotely access patient records through computer networks, passing the data to the required place in a few minutes or seconds. In the emergency, the information in the electronic medical record can be detected and displayed in the presence of the physician.

(2) Share. As we all know, the traditional paper medical records are very inconvenient and difficult when patients turn to other hospitals and need to check the diagnosis and treatment record of the previous hospital. This is not only a waste of valuable medical resources, but also increases unnecessary trouble for patients. The use of electronic medical records can overcome paper medical records deficiencies. The results of the diagnosis and treatment of the patients in each hospital can be transmitted through a computer network or a health card (photo card and IC card) carried by the patient to the hospital. The sharing of medical records will bring great convenience for medical treatment.

(3) Large storage. Because of computer storage technology, especially optical disc technology progress, storage capacity of the electronic medical record system database can be quite large.

(4) Convenience. Medical staff using electronic medical record system can conveniently store, retrieve replication and browse records, accurately carry out scientific research and statistical analysis, which greatly reduce the workload of manual collection and data entry and greatly improve the level of clinical research.

(5) Low cost. The electronic medical record system can reduce the expense of the patients and the expense of the hospital after one-time investment.

However, at present, there are some disadvantages of the electronic medical record. For example, a large number of computer hardware and software investment, personnel training, and some medical personnel difficult to adapt to computer operation. When the computer fails, it will cause the system to pause , therefore, it often needs to save the manual records. There are often various errors (mainly operational errors) when inputting medical records into a computer, which requires strict inspection to prevent errors and accidents.

8.4.3　Structure of Electronic Medical Record System

The electronic medical record usually supports patient data as a time sequence, information source and a record method. The structure of the case contains data, such as diagnosis, laboratory results and drug treatment. It is proved that the architecture information is very difficult, so the electronic medical record should firstly solve the structural problems. (An architecture knowledge driven medical record model is to be built and implemented an architecture data entry.) The basic data of the architecture data is that the input of the information that computer can understand and its characteristic is data with medical connotation.

Patient information includes the first page of medical records, medical, course records, nursing records, inspection results and hospital discharge records, and produces the diagnosis and treatment, inspection, operation, etc., a number of links in the subsystems for the system, its sources content is complex. In the electronic medical record system, information need to be organized as a whole according to the category and the time of occurrence, and it is needed to establish the structure of medical records. The structural data of the medical record information includes the structural data and the non-architecture data, such as nursing record and discharge record, etc. And system from the simple search query to complex judgment processing depends on information input and processing, so architecture medical record is the core problem.

Architecture electronic medical record is that from the point of medical informatics to natural language input mode of medical equipment in accordance with the requirements of medical terms architecture analysis, and these semantic structures eventually by the relational (object oriented) structure saved to the database. For example, the sentences description "abdominal pain for 2 days with vomiting disease", according to the categories of the words, it is divided into "abdominal" (noun), the "pain" (verb), "2" (numeral) and "day" (noun), "with vomiting" (verb) five parts. And "abdominal" is the word that describes the elements of the "body", and "pain" is the element description "symptoms", "2" is "numerical" elements, "day" is "time units" elements. Then we should find these elements in the appropriate element classification (assuming that the elements are defined).

One of the advantages of the electronic medical records is the convenience of the inter medical information exchange of medical records. In order to achieve this goal, it is needed to formulate the information exchange format and convert the medical records information into the standard exchange format, which can be transmitted or stored on the network.

Electronic medical records basic content should follow the HL7 standard selection function model. HL7 development of electronic medical record system function framework (FO) is composed of three parts: direct medical function (DC), support functional information (SP) and infrastructure capabilities (IN), which is used to summarize all the electronic medical record system functions (a total of 140). The functional paradigm (FP) only contains the electronic medical record system function to prepare. The functional paradigm must be constrained by the three components of the functional framework. (See Figure 8-4)

8.4.4   The Function of Electronic Medical Records

The multimedia electronic medical record system, was launched in 1994, it is a typical medical information system. The system is a set of images, video, audio and text in various multimedia miniature computer system, and it is from a variety of data sources and access information, Through a common desktop computer system medical staff can access to all the medical records of patients related, such as X-ray and ultrasound images, watch records relating

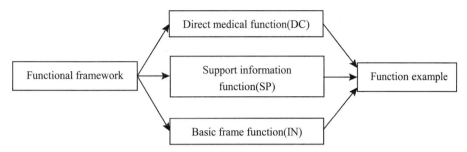

Figure 8-4   The Relationship Between Functional Framework and Functional Paradigm

to the condition of the video and audio. The multimedia electronic medical record system viewscope can connect with other medical information system and hospital information system.

The electronic medical record is the core of the hospital clinical information system. The main function of medical information system is to provide information service for the medical information service, and its function is to establish the medical records information for hospital. The main functions of the electronic medical record include ten aspects.

(1) Storage. With the electronic medical records as the core of the medical information system, the process of medical work will be a great change. If an emergency patient suddenly comes to the hospital, doctors can plugged patient health card into the computer, so that the computer will immediately show the patient's information, such as name, age, drug sensitivity and so on. At the time, according to the clinical manifestations of the patient, doctors will prescribe a check project. Information stored in the EMR system includes:

① Computer tomography (CT or CAT) images, nuclear magnetic resonance images, X-images, ultrasonic images and photos.

② Medical records, charts, letters and documents.

③ During the operation of the video recording and so on.

④ The relevant medical reports and the interpretation of the X-ray recording, etc.

(2) Medical Record Template Database.

① The patient's name, gender and other natural information.

② Patient admission, discharge, transfer, transfer and epidemic situation.

③ A variety of inspection records received by the patients.

④ A variety of treatment records for patients and doctors.

⑤ The nursing of the patient records.

(3) Automatic Detection and Incomplete Reminder.

In order to improve the quality of medical records and medical activities, and to assist the clinician to prevent medical errors, the system provides medical records of time limit monitoring function, give doctor online remind, and guidance of a doctor to complete records in time, such as which records should be completed first and which records can be completed later. At the same time, set the alarm line, such as the time remaining for the limit 8 hours, strengthen the warning to prevention of time limit deviation in the process of medical records.

(4) Support for a variety of medical special expressions (such as menstrual history, fetal heart, the location of the caries formula).

(5) Support the medical history document three grade examination function. After the completion of the examination, the doctors can immediately get the results of the examination and make a diagnosis and treatment advice. If it is difficult, the doctors can also ask superior doctors or specialist for consultation through computer network system. A superior physician or specialist may present consultation in his office or home to help the treatment plan for the doctor. The application of electronic medical record and computer information system will greatly shorten the time of medical consultation and improve the quality greatly.

(6) Support to modify the traces of retention, at all levels to retain the revised marks of doctors. Electronic medical records use word collection of patient information, with features of powerful editing and easy to use. However, it's free to modify the record, copy medical records and lack of quality control. In order to ensure the quality of medical records, to maintain the legitimate rights and interests of patients, electronic medical records must be kept revised marks in the medical records.

(7) Time control mechanism, technology of workflow, the task automatically prompt to remind the medical personnel according to the quality, quantity and complete medical record writing work, effectively avoid the lack of medical document writing and write leakage, delay writing.

(8) Support data element binding, achieve multi document synchronization refresh technology.

(9) Form processing ability (can facilitate the table records), support for tables nest and split cells, delete rows, columns to delete, add rows, adding a column, table insert elements, table width of manual or automatic adjustment.

(10) Support input numerical validity check. For example, when the doctor input the number which is invalidity, the system will feedback in time.

8.4.5   Case Study of Electronic Medical Record System

The main functions of the electronic medical record system should include creating the EMR function, patients with previous diagnosis and treatment information management function, hospital medical records management, orders management, examination and inspection report management function, electronic medical records show function, clinical knowledge base function, medical quality management function, electronic medical records system docking function, and so on.

8.4.5.1   Electronic Medical Record Creation Function

(1) Patient unique identification code. To create an electronic medical record for patients, the patient must be endowed with a unique and readable identity within the medical institution, and all electronic medical records of the patient must contain solely the identity information of the patient. Electronic medical record system supports the use of a unique identification number for all medical records of patients. The unique identification can be automatically generated by the system, but also by the manual allocation. This logo for patients and medical staff is readable, you can print on paper medical records, which facilitates the working effectiveness of medical personnel.

(2) Patient master index. The main index is created for each patient's electronic medical record. Patients record their basic information, including name, gender, birth date, address, contact number and others, and allow the main index information necessary to amend, supplement and improvement. Associated with unique identification code and the main index of patient's basic information, when patients do not carry or forget their own unique identification, medical staff can rely solely on the patient's basic information to identify patient's information. Other patient's information, such as medical records, medical insurance number, identity card number and other electronic medical records, must be associated with a unique identification number. In the actual business, it is easy for medical division to remember the patient's name, the number of beds that are used by nurses, hospital will utilize medicare card to position patients. The information in the system should be related to the unique identification code.

(3) The function of avoiding repeating. New electronic medical records, is the system that can automatically rely on the patient's name, gender and birth date to determine whether the patient has been in repetition and prompt patient to repeat the list. After further judgment and confirmation, the operator can decide to create a new medical record or not. The record repeating has become very common now, and the system according to the basic information of the patients, the provinces card data automatic detection and prompt the user may exist in the same patients with multiple copies of medical records of, after manual confirmation of duplicate records by modifying an identity to merge.

8.4.5.2   Patients with Past Diagnosis and Treatment Information Management

Previous diagnostic information is formed in patients with previous treatment process of medical records, including the patient's disease history, operation history, medication history, history of allergies, the previous investigation results. The above informations are important for doctors in the process of diagnosis and treatment. The electronic medical record system has the functions of adding, modifying, deleting, and so on.

Patient's history of allergy and adverse reactions directly affects the safety of medical treatment. When medical personnel prescribes, the system can utilize the patient's history of drug allergy and adverse reactions, giving the medical staff a warning to avoid medical errors. Allergic drug is not a specific drug, but a certain type of drug or drug composition requires an appropriate method to ensure electronic medical records system for automatic judgment.

8.4.5.3 Inpatient Medical Records Management

(1) Entry and editing of medical records. Electronic medical record system provides in-patient medical records double signature functions. Firstly, it needs the doctor's medical record writing practice, then it should get medical institutions registered physician reviewing and modifying, ensuring that the writers and reviewers and the double signature. When doctors confronted with a referral medical records, the system provides basic information of patients, medical information, auxiliary examination report query and other functions, and selects content directly into the medical record at the specified position. To provide a common terminology thesaurus auxiliary input function, the term lexicon, which is provided in the hospital medical records in embedded images, tables, multimedia data and editing functions, includes name and name of disease and drug. After the completion of the medical records and the confirmation of the preservation, the change and deletion of the medical records of the patient must be kept to the operation marks, and the electronic medical records created by the lower level medical personnel shall be permitted by the higher medical personnel.

(2) Medical record template management. Provide free text entry function; provide the function of the same information in the patient's medical record in the development of the medical records; provide a structured interface template. It automatically records the doctors to modify and delete the medical records, and the users to modify the function of management. Provides users with the functions of the user defined medical record template, and the use of the template to carry out the scope of the classification management functions. The use of medical record template includes creating individual, department and hospital. Figure 8-5 for the hospital medical record template interface.

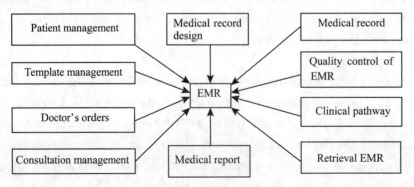

Figure 8-5   For the Hospital Medical Record Template Interface

（3）Nursing record management. Provide the function of the vital signs of the recorded patients, including body temperature, pulse, respiration and blood pressure; provide custom life signs, in clinical departments, according to different disease, specialist attention life signs and customization can be by clinical nursing staff to achieve the desired; provide operation nursing record of single input function, nursing information generating device provides interface data automatic acquisition to the corresponding project of nursing record of operation. In order to simplify the nurse entry, it provides a shared function with the physician to record the medical records, the doctor's advice and parts of the contents of the medical records.

8.4.5.4　Doctor's Orders Management

According to the type of medical activity, the doctor's advice can be divided into the types of medicine, examination, nursing, food and so on. In accordance with the duration and the number of execution, the doctors' advice can be divided into long-term and temporary medical advice, and long-term doctor's order is valid for more than 24 hours. According to the occasions, the doctor's advice can be divided into outpatient and hospital medical advice. Management is to the doctor's advice, delivery and execution of management. Figure 8-6 is the typical treatment process for a doctor's advice.

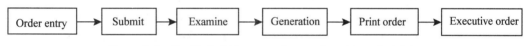

Figure 8-6　The Typical Treatment Process for a Doctor's Advice

8.4.5.5　Inspection Report Management

Inspection records are include ultrasound, radiology, nuclear medicine, endoscopy, pathology, ECG, etc., inspection records include clinical blood, body fluids, biochemistry, immunology, molecular biology, etc. The examination report is an objective reflection of the physiological and pathological conditions of the patients, which has important clinical value for the diagnosis and treatment of diseases. The electronic medical record system should ensure the doctors complete the report, the clinical departments of doctors and nurses on time, so as to improve the overall efficiency of medical institutions. Inspection and inspection report management function is mainly for all kinds of inspection, inspection report of the collection, modification, inform and check.

8.4.5.6　Electronic Medical Record Display

Electronic medical records in the way of visual, effective and convenient to show the patient's medical records and provide support for medical personnel comprehensive, effective control of medical records of patients, and in accordance with the sequence of hospitalization time, medical records classification finishing medical records, and in accordance with the basic information of the patients, visiting time, medical departments, disease coding information retrieval query function.

8.4.5.7   Clinical Knowledge Base

Clinical knowledge library physician prescribed and choice of treatment programs provide assistance, through active prompt or alarm and help doctors choose the right treatment, standardize the medical behavior. Clinical knowledge base can be classified into clinical pathway knowledge base, clinical diagnosis and treatment guideline, clinical database, rational use of knowledge base and medical insurance policy. To clinical pathway knowledge base as an example and need to provide according to the patient's condition is manually determined to enter the specific disease clinical pathway management function; provide clinical physician and path selection, to generate all kinds of orders and inspection functions on a single application; provide implementation clinical pathway, variation and for recording function.

8.4.5.8   Medical Quality Management and Control

Electronic medical records are in the capacity of comprehensive, timely collection and analysis of medical information, and provide a strong support for medical quality management. The real time analysis and supervision of patients medication orders can be found in the medical records of irrational use of drugs; analysis of the patient's test results, vital signs, treatment operation, medication and other information can be found potential infective enteritis; according to the disease surveillance of patients, medical expenses, can control unreasonable medical single disease; through the use of supervision for the high value consumables can supplies auxiliary judgment of irrational use.

8.4.5.9   Interface Function

Electronic medical record system should support the establishment of the data interface between the clinical departments and pharmacy management, examination and inspection, medical equipment management, management fees and other departments, and gradually realizes the data sharing and optimizes work flow, improves the work efficiency.

For example, the interface of pharmacy management system. Through drug orders or prescriptions sent to the pharmacy in real time, pharmacy staff can get the information in the shortest time, do a good job of medicine. If the selected drug is out of stock, it provides the same or similar pharmacological effect of the existing inventory, to avoid the drug insufficience caused the doctor's advice or prescription not act.

References

1. Alan D. Lopez, Colin D. Mathers. Global Burden of Disease and Risk Factors[M]. World Bank Publications, 2006.

2. Institute of Medicine. The Future of the Public's Health in the 21st Century[M]. Washington D.C.: The National Academy Press, 1988.

3. James A. Graham, Raymond L. Goldsteen, Karen Goldsteen, et al. Introduction to Public Health[M]. New York: Springer Publishing Company, 2010.

4. Liang Wannian. Health Service Management (3rd) [M]. Beijing: People's Medical Publishing House, 2007.

5. Lu Zuxun, Mao Zongfu. Social Medicine (3rd)[M]. Beijing: Science Press, 2009.

6. National Institutes of Health. The Burden of Digestive Diseases in the United States [M]. Createspace, 2014.

7. Sandra Dawson, Zoë Slote Morris. Future Public Health: Burdens, Challenges and Opportunities[M]. London: Palgrave Macmilian, 2009.

8. The National Health and Family Planning Commission. The 2015 China Health Statistical Yearbook (in Chinese)[R]. Beijing: Peking Union Medical College Press, 2015.

9. Widad Akrawi. Global Burden of Disease and Epidemiological Aspects[M]. Grin Verlag Publications, 2013.

10. WHO. World Health Report 2013: Research for Universal Health Coverage[R]. Geneva: WHO, 2013.

11. World Health Organization.The Global Burden of Disease 2004 Update [M].World Health Organization publication, 2008.

12. David Royse, Bruce A. Thyer, Deborah K. Padgett. Program Evaluation: An Introduction. Cengage Learning, 2013.

13. Louis Rowitz. Public Health Leadership. Burlington MA: Jones & Bartlett Publishers, 2013.